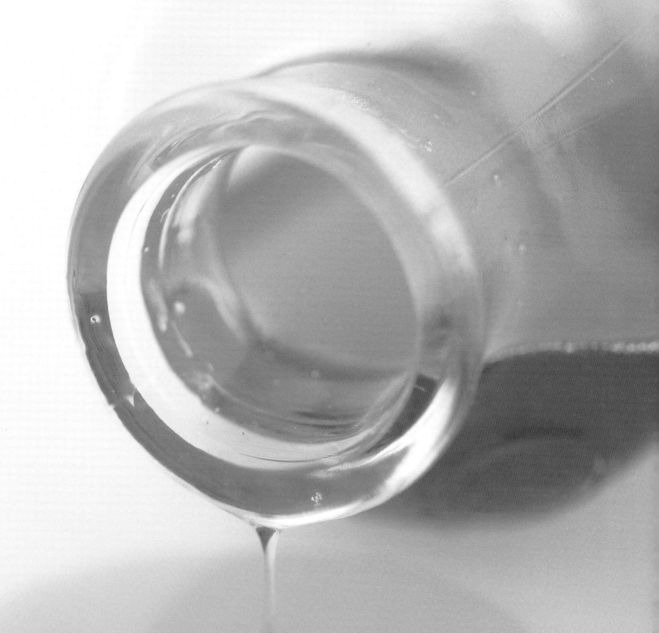

hand
&foot
massage

To Jenny Buckley and Gabriella Kispal
– with affection and respect

THIS IS A CARLTON BOOK

Text copyright © 2001 Mary Atkinson
Design copyright © 2001 Carlton Books Limited

First published by the Carlton Publishing Group 2001
20 Mortimer Street
London
W1T 3JW

A CIP catalogue record for this book is available from the British Library.

ISBN 1 84222 113 2

Art direction: Diane Spender
Design: Michael Spender
Commissioning Editor: Claire Richardson
Production: Alastair Gourlay
Photography: John Davis

Printed in Dubai

mary atkinson

hand &foot massage

massage taken to the extremes

photography by John Davis

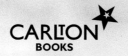
CARLTON
BOOKS

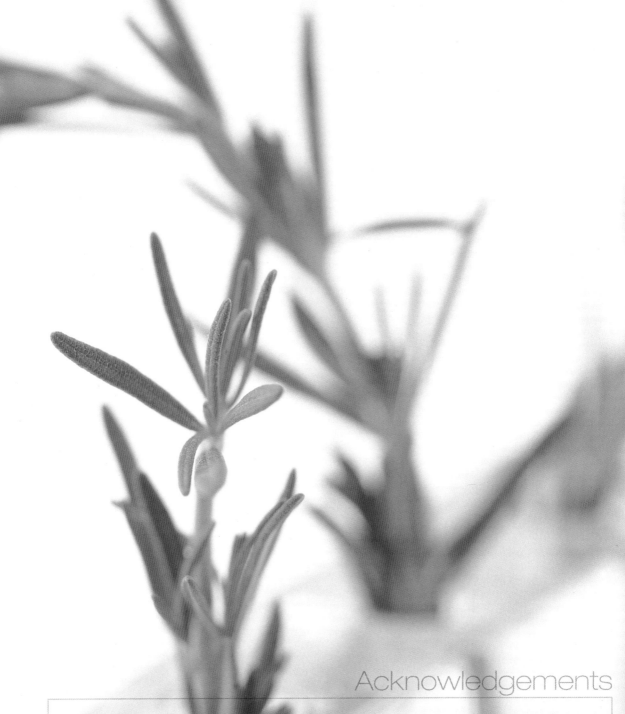

Acknowledgements

Grateful thanks to Jo Hammond and Anne Bennett, my massage tutors, who gave me the confidence and inspiration to embark on this project. Also to Frances Foster a very special clinical aromatherapist, who shared her expertise. My appreciation to Nina Guilfoyle, who helped me devise some of the massage routines – and to Peter, Stephen, Sarah, Richard, Emma and Lizzie for lending me their hands and feet! I would also like to thank my agent, Chelsey Fox, for her determination, Allyson Bettridge and Susie Jennings for their constant encouragement, and Bernadette Cassidy for her useful comments. And last, but by no means least, my special thanks to all the team at Carlton Books and my talented editor, Richard Emerson.

Contents

Massage is a wonderful way of saying "Thank you" to

your hands and feet for all the relentless work they do.

All too often we take our hands and feet for granted. It

is only when something goes wrong that we realize just

how much we depend on them for everyday activities.

Benefits
of a caring touch

Regular care – through massage, manicure and pedicure – can prevent many common problems arising, make hands and feet look more attractive and bring far-reaching benefits for emotional and physical health and well-being.

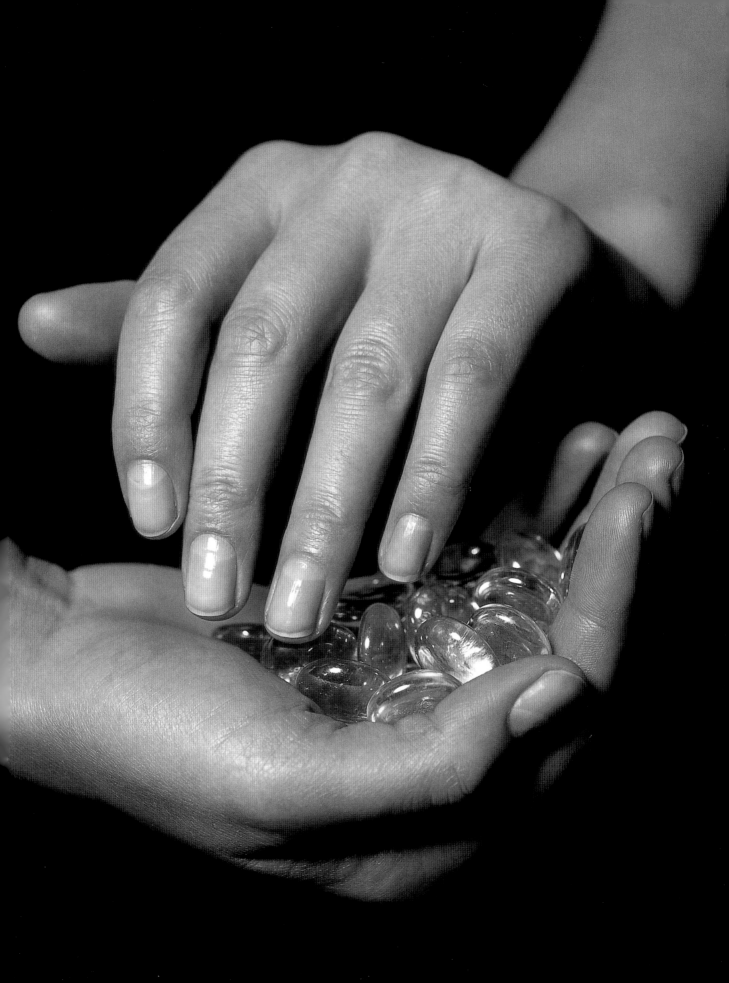

Soothe or stimulate

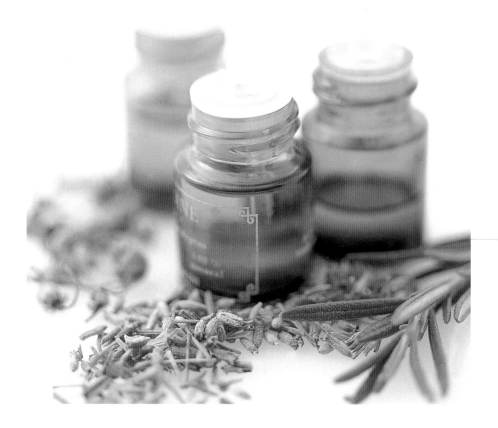

H ands help us to communicate with others and express our creativity. Yet we reward them by soaking them in strong detergents and exposing them to the harshest of weather. Feet enable us to walk, run and jump for joy. Yet we cram them into ill-fitting shoes and expect them to bear our full body weight for hours on end. It is no wonder that skin becomes dry, hard and cracked, joints start to stiffen and ache, and the blood circulation to the extremities slows down, leading to cold and painful fingers and toes. Hands and feet deserve care and attention – and respond surprisingly quickly to a therapeutic touch. The palms of the hands and soles of the feet contain thousands of sensory nerve endings, making them among the most sensitive areas of the body. Massage can be used to stimulate or calm the whole being.

Hand and foot massage can be effective in relieving tiredness after a long day, or relaxing an irritable child during a difficult time. It can refresh and revitalize, or soothe and nurture. Once you have learnt a few basic techniques, you can use massage in many different situations – from sitting in a cramped aeroplane seat to relaxing in your own front room – for yourself and others, children and adults.

The healing properties of massage have been recognized for many centuries. Hieroglyphics show that wealthy Egyptians received a daily massage with fragrant oils to help protect their skin from the drying effects of the desert sun. The Romans enjoyed a therapeutic massage at the end of their regular bathing routine while, in India, massage with aromatic oils and spices is an integral part of the ancient holistic system of Ayurvedic medicine. However, the tremendous boom in technology has rather overshadowed the benefits of natural therapy and it is only in recent years that a demand for massage has re-emerged.

Advantages of hand and foot massage

The hands and feet offer the perfect introduction to massage – both for the giver and the receiver. They are very accessible – so they can be massaged just about anywhere, anytime. You do not even have to move from your favourite armchair! There is no need for any special equipment and the only expense is a little cream or oil. Nor does a simple hand or foot massage have to take up a great deal of time to be effective – indeed, it has been estimated that just a ten minute massage is sufficient to induce a good night's sleep. And the real bonus for many people is that there are no concerns about the embarrassment or inconvenience of undressing.

note

This book is not a substitute for formal teaching but will introduce you to some of the basic techniques and encourage you to develop your own personal style of hand and foot massage.

checklist

Benefits of hand and foot massage

The therapeutic effects of hand and foot massage last long after the treatment is over. The short and long term benefits are individual, varied and cumulative and include the following:

- Relief from pain and stiffness in the muscles, tendons and ligaments of the hands and feet.
- Increased mobility of the joints in the hands and feet.
- Improved blood circulation to nourish and warm the extremities.
- More efficient removal of waste products and excess fluid to reduce puffiness.
- Strengthened immune system to fight infection.
- Opportunity to enjoy time to unwind and relax away from everyday stresses and hassles.
- A sense of tranquillity, calmness and enhanced well-being.
- Improved skin and nail condition and colour.
- Increased self-esteem and self-worth.
- Psychological comfort when emotions are in turmoil and words seem futile.
- Bonding – a way of expressing "I'm here for you" in difficult times.
- Greater awareness of the need to look after hands and feet, which can help prevent many common hand and foot disorders from occurring.

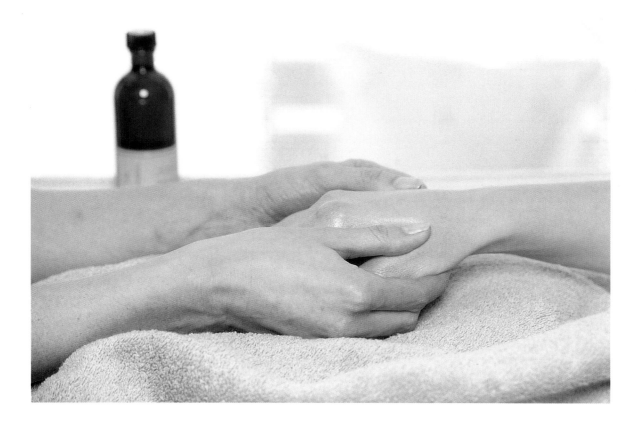

Increasingly, health care professionals are waking up to the benefits of hand and foot massage for children and adults. For one thing, it is often more practical than body massage for ill, elderly and frail people. Trained therapists, nurses and volunteers offer massage in hospitals, hospices and nursing homes where time and space are often limited. Relatives and friends, who might otherwise be unsure how they can help a loved one during an illness, or through childbirth, have found that giving a hand or foot massage can be a valuable way of showing love and support.

Looking and feeling good

Hand and foot massage helps to relieve muscular tension and fatigue that so often builds up through repetitive movements or after holding one position for a long time. It eases stiffness and discomfort in the joints, stimulates blood circulation and drains away toxins to encourage healthy skin and nails. The pleasure of a pampering, caring touch triggers the release of endorphins, the body's natural painkillers, leading to a sense of deep relaxation and well-being. Numerous studies have shown that a simple hand or foot massage can bring significant relief from emotional stress and reduce anxiety levels.

Above all, hand and foot massage provides the time to stop whatever you are doing for a few minutes and simply be still and quiet. This healing period in the day allows space for much-deserved "me" time to help you unwind from the stresses and strains of everyday life. It offers an opportunity to reflect and focus, and enables you to look at life from a new perspective. People often emerge from the relaxing experience of a hand or foot massage with a greater sense of responsibility for their own health, which in turn boosts their self-esteem and self-respect.

Regular massage, especially when complemented by manicure, pedicure and general care, will improve the condition of hands and nails – often the first areas to reveal the tell-tale signs of ageing. Nourishing oils and creams help keep skin soft and supple, and maintain nail strength and shine. And once you notice the difference, you will enjoy a new awareness of the need to respect your hard-working hands and feet. When they look and feel good, so do you!

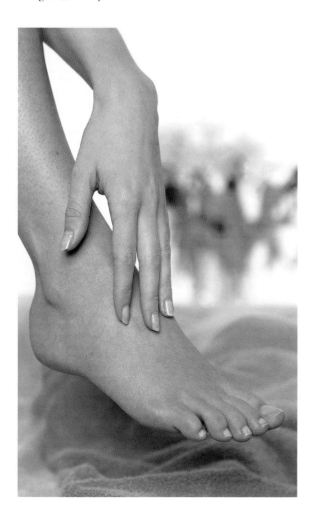

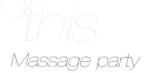

try this

Massage party

For her thirtieth birthday, Jennifer decided to plan a party with a difference. She organized a girls' night in for eight of her friends – with some massage oils and candles! "It was the best party ever," she enthuses. "I arranged the room so that it looked restful and put on the answerphone so that we would not be disturbed. Then we all took off our shoes and socks, and massaged each other's feet.

"Everyone was very giggly at first, and we all kept saying how much we hated our feet, but we soon calmed down. We got into pairs and one did the massage while the other sat back and relaxed. Then we moved around so that we were in a different two-some for the next massage.

"We experimented as we went along – using our instinct to stroke and rub, and working out which moves felt the best. We all had our own likes and dislikes. One of my friends said she was concerned because she had ticklish feet, but she was pleased that the massage was firm and didn't make them tickle. While we were massaging, there was an atmosphere of trust in the room and we all felt a wonderful release of worries and hassles.

"I felt great afterwards – a real sense of inner peace and well-being. And I had a brilliant night's sleep. My friends said the same – we all want to make our foot massage evenings a regular event."

An understanding of the positive effects of massage on our physical and psychological health can help you adapt your sequence of movements to ensure maximum benefits for yourself and your massage partner.

Hands and feet
– inside and out

Before you begin to massage hands and feet it is important to appreciate how they form an integral part of the whole body and cannot be viewed in isolation from the systems and structures that make up each individual person.

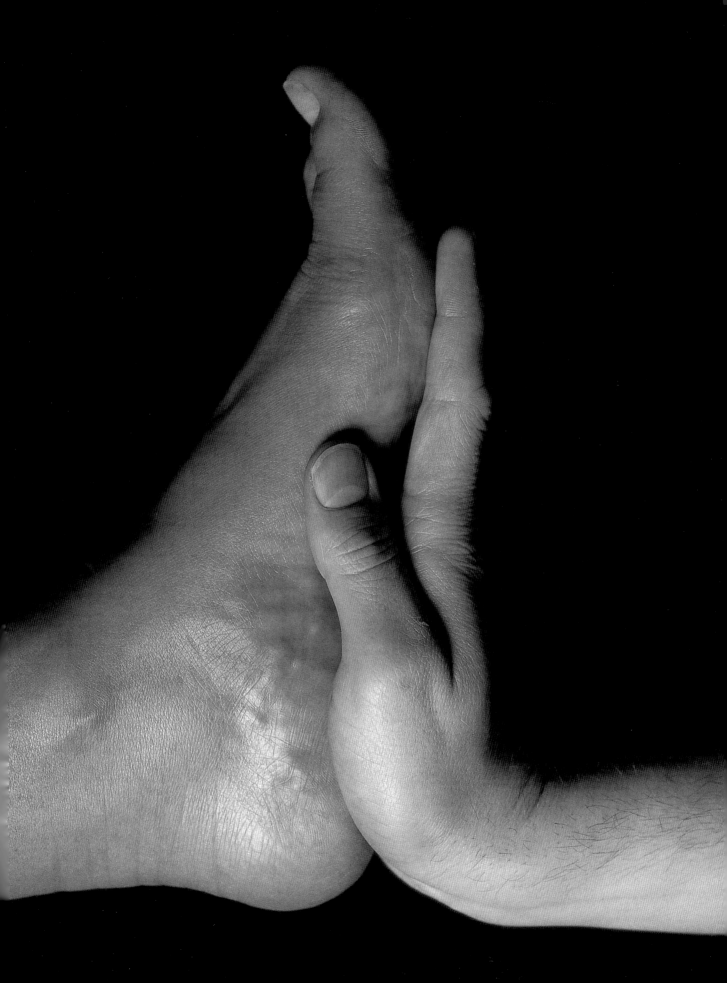

The relaxation response

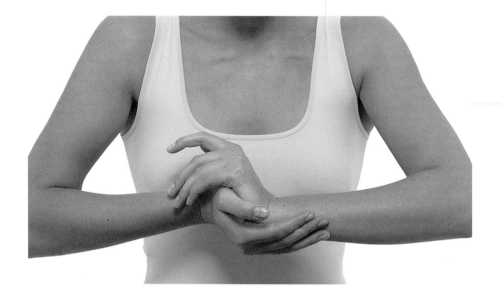

One of the most valuable benefits of massage is deep physical and mental relaxation – which is becoming increasingly necessary in our modern stress-filled lives. When you are faced with a stressful situation, whether real or perceived, the alarm bell sounds and the body responds by secreting hormones including adrenalin and cortisol to prepare for instant action. This "fight or flight" response is a primitive survival tactic to cope with a purely physical threat, such as an attack from a wild animal.

Muscles tense for optimum performance, either in facing the attacker or making an instant get-away. The heart and lungs work extra hard to speed up the flow of blood and oxygen to the muscles and brain. Blood pressure and pulse rate rise. Breathing quickens.Blood is diverted from the skin (causing it to go white) and the stomach (leading to the sensation of "butterflies") to provide the muscles and brain with extra energy supplies. Short bouts of stress, such as a white-knuckle ride at a theme park, can be exhilarating – indeed, beneficial for health and well-being.

However, when stress is prolonged over days, months and years, it puts the mind and body in a constant state of "overdrive" and saps your mental and physical energy. The effects often creep up so slowly that many people don't notice the changes within themselves. If allowed to continue, chronic stress can lead to permanently raised blood pressure, digestive disorders, migraine, back pain, heart disease and skin complaints. Stress hormones also depress the immune system, leading to greater susceptibility to diseases.

fact

Around 70% of all illness is believed to be directly or indirectly associated with mental and emotional stress.

How massage helps our mood

Hand and foot massage work on physical and psychological levels simultaneously, countering physical and mental tension and encouraging well-being.

- As physical aches and pains are eased by massage, so it becomes easier to adopt a calmer, more positive frame of mind and cope better with daily hassles and worries.
- During a massage, there is an opportunity to sit quietly and allow the mind and body time to relax and recharge. The pleasure of caring, physical contact helps boost self-esteem and encourages the release of "feel good" chemicals called endorphins that help fight pain, lift your mood and – by counteracting stress – allowing the immune system to fight infection.
- Deep physical and mental relaxation induced by massage has been shown to help lower blood pressure, slow down breathing and relieve early symptoms of stress, thus preventing more serious longer-term health problems.
- Suppressed emotions may be released, so bringing emotional relief. The relaxation effect encourages deep breathing, which relaxes the body and calms the mind.

- The immediate benefits of a hand or foot massage bring an increased sense of self-awareness, which often leads to early recognition of stress signals and the realization of the need for mental and physical relaxation in everyday life.
- Regular gentle massage of arthritic hands can ease pain and improve mobility in the fingers – enabling them to hold a cup to drink, for example – thereby helping to increase a person's independence and reducing emotional stress.

The circulatory systems

The healthy circulation of blood is essential to the vitality of all the bodily systems. Blood carries supplies of oxygen and nutrients, such as minerals, vitamins and glucose, to the billions of living cells within the body enabling them to produce the energy needed to fuel the thousands of chemical activities essential to life. During the process of releasing and using energy, known as cell metabolism, various waste products, such as carbon dioxide and water, are released into tiny blood vessels, called capillaries, and into the spaces between the cells. Blood drains away these metabolic wastes and other impurities so they do not accumulate in the tissues.

The blood circulatory system is assisted by the lymphatic system, an intricate network of glands, vessels and tubes that extends throughout the whole body, removing viruses, bacteria and other foreign materials, fighting infection, and draining excess fluid from tissue spaces. Any impurities are carried in a liquid, known as lymph, which travels through the lymphatic system, passing through several lymph nodes (sometimes known as lymph "glands") where it is cleansed and filtered, before eventually draining into the bloodstream.

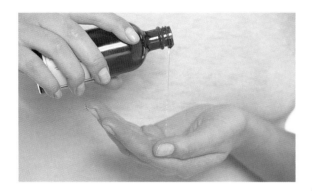

How massage helps our circulatory systems

Massage stimulates the blood and lymphatic systems. This brings a number of benefits to the tissues of the hands and feet:

- A more efficient blood flow ensures a steady supply of oxygen and nutrients to the living cells of the body, so aiding their proper functioning and stimulating cell growth, division, renewal and healing.
- The speedier removal of carbon dioxide, metabolic waste and excess fluid helps improve the condition of skin and nails, and also prevents stiffness, pain and any puffiness in ankles, feet, wrists and hands.
- The increased supply of blood generates heat in cold hands and feet. This encourages general relaxation and aids the absorption of small amounts of oil through the skin.
- A more efficient lymphatic system helps prevent and fight general infections, including those affecting the hands and feet (see page 120).

The outer covering

The skin is one of nature's finest works of art. This complex organ, the largest in the body, provides a highly flexible protective covering. It gives us shape and holds us together. Skin keeps the body fluids in and acts as a first line of defence to shield the internal structures and systems from injury and invasion by unwanted visitors such as dirt, bacteria, fungi and viruses. Although it is largely waterproof, it allows some absorption of water and substances such as pure essential oils. The skin has three main layers, the epidermis, the dermis, and the subcutaneous, or "below the skin", layer each with a different composition and function.

fact

The blood circulation through the skin can, when necessary, increase by up to 150 times, to increase heat loss from the skin.

Epidermis

The top skin layer is called the epidermis and is the one that can be seen and touched. This is the layer where cell renewal takes place. The epidermis is made up of millions of cells that are constantly growing and replacing themselves. The epidermis is, itself, made up of different layers. The lowest one, the basal layer, is where new skin cells form. It takes around 27 days for cells to move up through the epidermal layers. As they do so, they fill with a tough protein material called keratin and slowly flatten out and die. Once they reach the surface of the skin they get rubbed off, usually through contact with clothes and other surfaces. As old cells are shed, fresh ones take their place, and so the cycle continues. If the dead cells are allowed to accumulate, they can make the skin dry, hard and dull.

fact

Skin produces a pigment known as melanin to offer some protection from the harmful rays of the sun. However, it cannot deal with "over" exposure – which can lead to age spots and a leathery appearance. So always protect your skin during sunny weather.

Dermis

The dermis lies directly underneath the epidermis and its main function is to support and nourish the epidermis and other skin structures. The dermis contains blood and lymph vessels, nerve endings, sweat and sebaceous (oil) glands and hair follicles.

- Sensory nerve endings in the skin provide essential information about the surroundings. They are extremely sensitive to heat, cold, damage, light touch and deep pressure and respond to specific stimuli by giving feedback to the brain.
- Sweat glands play a major role in removing excess heat and toxic waste products from the body – via sweat that seeps through the pores. Sweat glands respond to factors such as heat, exercise and emotional and hormonal changes. The feet have around 250,000 sweat glands – more than any other part of the body – so it's hardly surprising that many people suffer from damp and sweaty feet. It has been estimated that, on average, the foot loses around a quarter of an egg cup of fluid every day.
- Sebaceous glands secrete an oily fluid known as sebum. Sebum is a natural moisturizer, helping to keep the skin soft and supple. When these glands are underactive, which often occurs in older people, it leads to dry skin that may become very thin or flaky, and more susceptible to injury and infection. Sebum also helps keep the skin waterproof and combines with sweat to create an acidic coating to guard against the growth of bacteria and fungi. Immersing hands or feet in extremely hot water or using harsh soaps and chemicals can upset this natural protective coating. Sebaceous glands are found on most areas of the body, but there are none on the palms of the hands or soles of the feet.

Fatty layer

The subcutaneous layer lies beneath the dermis and contains adipose tissue, where fat is stored. The subcutaneous layer helps reduce heat loss through the skin and also acts as a protective cushion for underlying structures, as well as providing a reserve store of fat for energy.

Skin thickness

Skin varies in thickness over the body. The thinnest part is around the eyes, where it is only 0.5 mm (1/50 in) thick. The thickest part is on the palms of the hands and soles of the feet where it is around 6 mm (1/4 in) thick. Indeed, hands and feet have an extra layer of skin, which is covered in ridges designed to stop them slipping. These ridges are arranged in patterns that form each person's own distinctive fingerprint.

Healthy nails

Nails are designed to protect the delicate skin on fingers and toes from damage, and also enable you to do a wide variety of tasks. Finger and toe nails grow from the dermis, which is richly supplied with blood and lymph vessels. This ensures that nutrients and oxygen are delivered

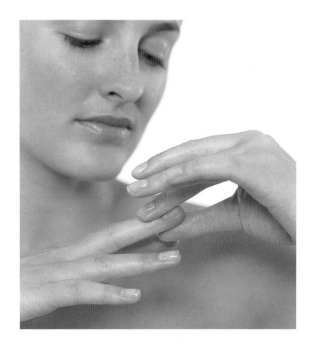

to the cells of the developing nail, and that waste products are speedily removed. The nail is attached to an area of tissue known as the nail bed. The light pinkish colour of a healthy nail is due to the blood vessels underneath, which provide nourishment. The nail only becomes white when it is detached from the nail bed.

A nail is formed by living cells that accumulate at the matrix (or nail root) at the base of the visible nail, and continually multiply. As these cells grow upward toward the protruding, or free edge, they fill with the tough and durable protein keratin that makes nails, hair and skin so hardwearing. The visible nail, known as the nail plate, is made up of thin layers of keratin held together by oil and moisture to maintain resilience. The curved white area beneath the nail, known as the lunula, or half moon, is the only part of the matrix that can be seen. The cuticle, the pliable ridge of skin just above the matrix, is designed to protect the growing base of the nail from injury or infection by sealing off the opening between skin and nail. If the matrix is damaged this can lead to deformity of the nail.

Finger nails grow at around twice the speed of toenails. In an adult, it takes around six months for a healthy nail to grow from the cuticle to the free edge, but around 12 months for a toenail to do so. Growth decreases with age, largely due to the slowing down of the blood circulation to the developing nail cells. Finger nails grow faster on the hand that you use most – probably because the increased movement stimulates blood circulation.

fact

Nails grow faster in the summer, when ultra-violet rays from the sun tend to stimulate cell division, and slower in the winter, when circulation tends to become more sluggish.

How massage helps the skin

Hand or foot massage has many beneficial effects on the condition, texture and appearance of the skin and nails.

- Massage boosts blood and lymph circulation, thus speeding up the supply of nourishment and oxygen to the living, growing cells, and removing impurities and excess tissue fluid. This helps provide the ideal environment for cell growth, renewal, repair and division to ensure healthy skin and nails.
- The friction of the hands combined with improved blood circulation leads to an increase in the shedding of dead skin cells, a process known as desquamation, so helping prevent skin from becoming dry and hard.
- The sebaceous glands are stimulated to produce more sebum, which keeps the skin soft and supple and helps offer protection from infection.
- The sweat glands are also stimulated, which assists in the removal of waste products and helps prevent the pores getting clogged with dirt and dead skin cells.

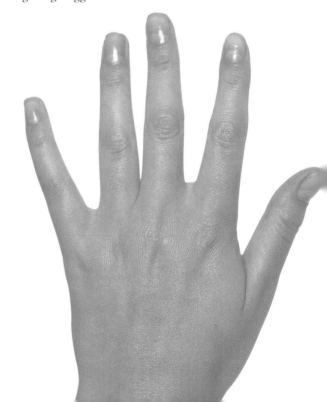

- Massage with a moisturizing cream or oil can keep the skin well lubricated and prevent excessively dry skin becoming sore and splitting.

Muscles, bones and other structures

Hands and feet are capable of an amazing variety of movements. This efficiency is entirely due to a highly sophisticated structure of bones, muscles, and other structures, such as the ligaments and tendons in the wrist, hand, ankle and foot. These work together to enable us to control movements as complicated as walking and jumping or writing and painting. Bones form the body's framework offering support and shape to structures such as hands and feet. Where movable bones meet they form joints. Different types of joint allow varying degrees of movement.

Muscles and tendons

Muscles are attached to bones on either side of a joint by fibres of tough connective tissue, known as tendons. Muscles exert a pull on the tendon, which moves the bone and any weight it is carrying. Muscles and tendons work in pairs to facilitate movement. One set of muscles and tendons acts to raise a bone, while the other set relaxes to allow the movement to take place – and vice versa. Tendons come in several different shapes. The tendons in the hands and feet are long and enclosed by slippery synovial sheaths, which enable them to slide when the fingers or toes bend. As we grow older, tendons and ligaments tend to shorten and tighten, which leads to stiffness and poor mobility.

Ligaments

Bones are bound together at joints by extremely strong bands of fibrous tissue known as ligaments. The ligaments bend as the joint bends, but as they only have limited ability to stretch they are able to prevent excessive movement between two bones. The term "double-jointed" means that in some people the ligaments can stretch more than usual and thus allow a greater range of movement.

Muscles and blood supply

Muscles have their own blood and lymphatic vessels. As the muscle relaxes, oxygenated blood flows in to nourish the tissues; as the muscle contracts, deoxygenated blood is forced out, carrying away impurities and metabolic waste products. If muscles are over-worked or tense, the local blood and lymph circulations are impeded, which leads to a shortage of oxygen and a build-up of waste products. This situation adversely affects the efficiency of the muscle, leading to muscle fatigue, soreness, discomfort, aching and transient pain.

Muscles and bones of the hand

The hand is a wonderfully versatile structure. It is strong enough to grasp and carry heavy objects, yet is capable of the precision and flexibility needed to make highly involved movements, such as writing or turning a door handle. Each hand is made up of 27 bones. There are:

- Eight carpals, which are irregularly shaped, and placed in two rows of four to form the wrist.
- Five metacarpals, which extend from the wrist to the fingers and make up the palm of the hand. The metacarpal in the thumb is the most mobile.
- Fourteen phalanges – two in the thumb and three in each of the fingers.

fact

Humans and other primates are the only creatures who can make a pinching movement, with the finger and thumb working independently.

The forearm is made up of two long bones – the radius and the ulna – which stretch from the elbow and work with the bones of the wrist to allow a wide range of movement.

There are few muscles in the hand itself. Some muscles lie on the outer edge of the palm and at the base of the thumb. Small muscles between the metacarpal bones enable the fingers to move from side to side. But the main muscles used in hand movements are situated in the forearm and connected to the fingers by long tendons. Muscles in the lower arm enable the palm to turn upward or downward, the wrist to rotate and the fingers and thumbs to curl and straighten. Movement is aided by joints, or knuckles, in the fingers and thumb, which help make the hand so flexible.

Tendons are attached at one end to the arm muscles and at the other to bones in the fingers and thumb. When the appropriate muscles contract, they pull on the tendons and so bend or stretch the fingers or thumb. The tendons are bound to the wrist by a strong ligament just above the wrist joint.

Try this out

To watch the tendons in action, place your hand palm down on a flat surface. Now raise your fingers and thumb. You will be able to see the five tendons along the back of the hand working to straighten your fingers. To see the reverse action, hold your hand out with your palm facing upward. Pull your sleeve back so you can see your forearm. Move your fingers toward the palm, one by one. Again, you will be able to see tendons working to close the fingers.

Muscles and bones of the foot

The foot supports the weight of the body and acts as a powerful lever to move the body forward when walking or running on different surfaces. The foot, combined with other senses, also helps us to maintain balance. These tasks are facilitated by a complex arrangement of bones, ligaments, tendons and muscles. The bones of the foot are positioned in a similar lay-out to those of the hand but the foot is a stronger and less flexible structure. The foot is made up of 26 bones. There are:

- Seven tarsals, which are irregularly shaped bones forming the ankle. The largest tarsal, the calcaneus, makes up the heel.
- Five metatarsals, which stretch between the ankle and the toes, and form the body of the foot. The metatarsal on the inside of the foot is the thickest and strongest, carrying the most body weight.
- Fourteen phalanges – two in the big toe and three in each of the other toes.

The bones and joints of the foot are arranged to form dynamic arches – two along the length of the foot, and one across the foot – between the ball of the foot and the heel. If you look at a footprint made by a normal, healthy foot you will see that only the outside of the foot touches the ground. The arches of the foot, which are maintained by strong ligaments and muscles, support the foot, absorb shock and provide leverage when walking, running and jumping. The height of the arches determines the shape of the foots. When the muscles and ligaments become strained and stretched, the arches may begin to weaken, which eventually leads to a condition known as "flat feet" (see page 122).

The lower leg is made up of the two long bones – the tibia and the fibula – which work with the bones of the ankle to allow a wide range of movement in the foot.

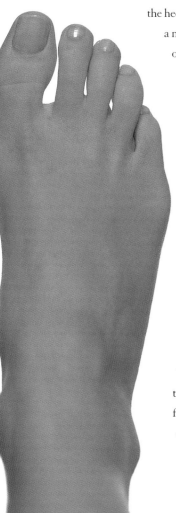

There are few muscles in the foot. The main muscles are in the sole of the foot and help to bend and spread the toes. The big toe is controlled by its own muscle as it plays such an important role in walking and maintaining balance. Small muscles on the top of the foot straighten and lift the toes. The main muscles are connected to the bones of the foot by long tendons. The ankle joint is supported by strong ligaments. When the appropriate muscles contract, they pull on the tendons and so stretch or bend the foot and toes. Muscles at the front of the leg help bend the foot upward at the ankle and straighten the toes; while muscles at the back of the leg lift the heel upward and curl the toes downward.

The Achilles tendon, situated at the back of the heel, is the strongest tendon in the whole body. It is attached at one end to the calf (gastrocnemius) muscle and at the other to the calcaneus, the largest bone in the foot, which forms the heel. This thick tendon is clearly seen when you stand on tiptoe or point your toes.

How massage helps muscles, tendons and ligaments

Hand and foot massage can help promote the health, strength and flexibility of muscles, tendons and ligaments.

- The increased flow of blood and lymph brings fresh supplies of nutrients and oxygen to muscles and joints and removes waste products and excess fluid. This helps improve joint mobility and reduces the stiffness, tiredness and aches so often caused by standing or long periods of repetitive hand movements.
- The increased blood supply and frictional heat creates warmth in the area which encourages relaxation, so bringing pain relief.

Taking time to select the most suitable oil or cream will enhance the benefits, and add considerably to the pleasure, of giving and receiving a hand or foot massage. Oils and creams act as a lubricant between your hands and the recipient's skin, so enabling a smoother, more fluent and effective massage without dragging or stretching the skin.

Oils and Creams
for massage

Carefully chosen emollients also support the health-giving benefits of massage by moisturizing, strengthening and protecting the skin. These creams and oils can also be combined with aromatic pure essential oils to have a relaxing or stimulating effect on mind and body.

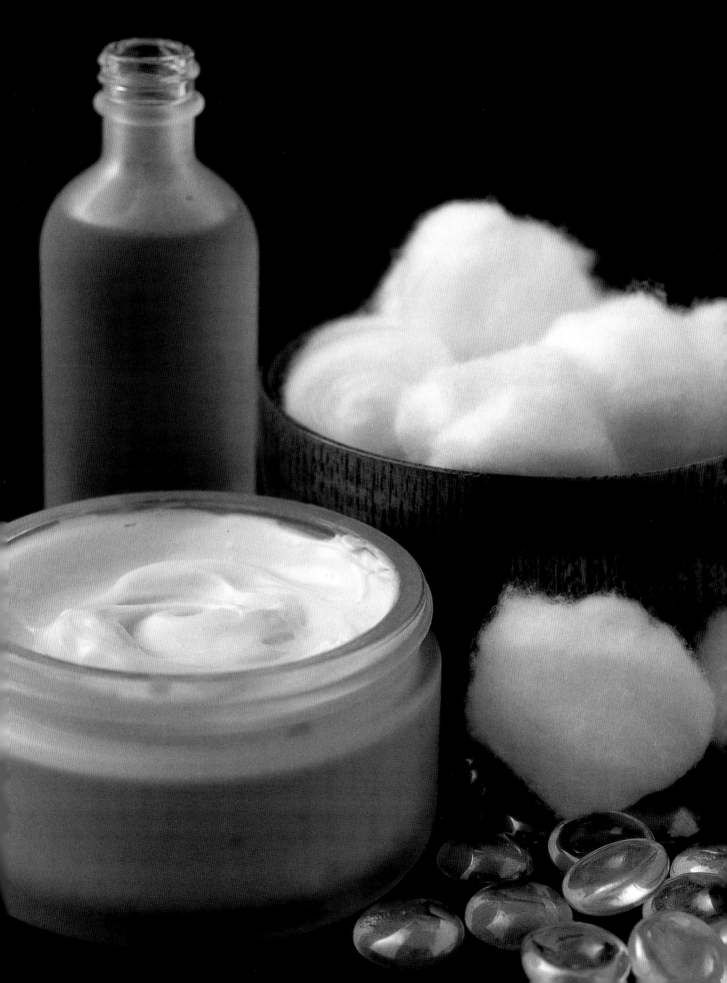

Choosing a massage medium

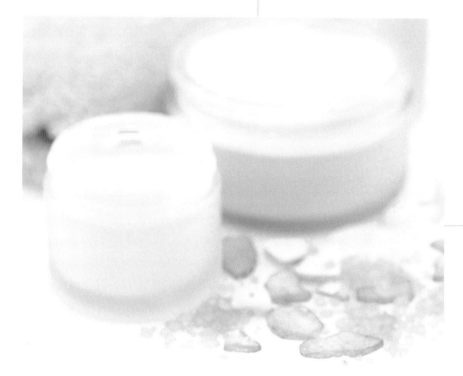

There is a wide variety of oils and creams that are ideal lubricants for hand and foot massage. Indeed, the choice can seem quite bewildering at first. Chemists, supermarkets and health food stores all stock a selection of ready-blended hand and foot massage mediums created to suit individual skin texture or match the mood of the occasion. Or you may prefer to follow the wisdom of past generations by blending your own creams and oils, using natural ingredients and adding pure essential oils to give that all-important personal touch to the massage. It is worth experimenting with different massage oils and creams to discover those that are the most effective and enjoyable to use. You may well find that your massage partner has particular preferences too.

Oils versus creams

Massage oils are readily available and highly versatile. They help soften and nourish the skin and provide a good "slip" so your hands can flow smoothly from one movement to the next. However, men with very hairy skin find massage using oil can be quite painful as the hairs tend to get pulled. Some people also dislike the sticky feel of oil on their skin after a massage – so it is useful to have a towel ready to wipe off the excess, or you could even use cologne. Oil tends to stain, so make sure that it does not spill on your massage partner's clothes.

Many people find creams easier to use than oils. They give an excellent slip and can help facilitate a deep, firm massage. They are particularly beneficial for very dry skin as they tend to stay on the skin surface longer than oils, allowing more time for the top layers of skin to absorb the nourishment. Use a rich non-medicated cream especially designed for massage. Ordinary vanishing or moisturizing creams and lotions are absorbed so quickly that you need to keep applying more, which disturbs the flow of the massage.

Buying ready blended creams and oils

Commercial blended oils and creams can provide a good starting point for hand and foot massage. Many brands have pretty packaging or boast special benefits – but be cautious. They do vary greatly in texture and quality, however, so buy in small quantities from a reputable retailer and test a selection. Be sure the oil or cream has a pleasant aroma and feels smooth on your hands. Some commercial blends smell synthetic, others may leave a sticky residue on your hands and on the skin of your massage partner, or may be too thin in texture to slide easily over the skin.

Natural vegetable oils

Choose a natural vegetable oil such as sweet almond oil, which can be used on its own, or combined with other base oils or pure essential oils. Look for oils that are unrefined and free from additives. It is best to buy cold pressed oils (look on the label) as oils that have been extracted through heating, as in vegetable cooking oil, have much of their nourishing properties destroyed. If possible, select organic oils as these have been produced without the use of chemical fertilizers or pesticides. Health food stores, some large supermarkets, large pharmacies and aromatherapy mail order catalogues are good sources for buying good quality base oils. Most natural vegetable oils last around six months before turning rancid and becoming unsuitable for massage – so avoid buying in bulk. Store in a cool, dry place, out of direct sunlight.

Natural massage creams

You can make your own massage cream, using pure, natural ingredients, or buy an unfragranced cream base and add pure essential oils. Many health food stores and aromatherapy mail order catalogues offer a selection of base creams and ingredients so you can create your own. Most base creams are made from a combination of natural ingredients including beeswax, pure vegetable oils and a preservative such as vitamin E. Base creams containing a preservative usually last around six months before becoming unsuitable for massage. Store in a cool, dry place out of direct sunlight.

note

If you or your massage partner have an allergy to nuts, you may prefer to avoid nut oils. Although there is no proven evidence that nut oils cause an allergic reaction, you may wish to minimize the risk.

Pure essential oils

Despite the name, essential oils are quite different from vegetable oils. They are non-greasy, volatile and characterized by an individual fragrance. Essential oils are concentrated chemicals derived from different parts of a living plant – bark, flower, leaf, petal, fruit, gum or root. Indeed, different parts of the same plant can produce different essential oils, each with their own specific and very powerful chemical mix. Over the years, hundreds of different essential oils have been discovered which, when used correctly by a trained aromatherapist, can have a therapeutic effect on mind, body and emotions. Some essential oils are safe for home use, provided they are treated with great care and respect. As a general rule, most essential oils should never be applied directly to the skin – lavender and tea tree oils are exceptions. For a massage, essential oils are used in minute quantities and combined with vegetable oils or base creams to be applied to the skin. The essential oils dissolve easily and completely in the lubricant. This acts as a carrier to allow the oils to be absorbed through the skin layers and taken into the blood stream, where they can travel around the body fulfilling different healing functions. The distinctive aromas of pure essential oils are also inhaled and can have a profound influence on moods – for example, certain scents can relax, invigorate or uplift.

Essential oils are sold in health food stores, pharmacies and through aromatherapy mail-order outlets. A qualified aromatherapist will be able to suggest a reputable supplier. However, it is important to buy with care – a pure essential oil can enter the body within twenty minutes and may stay in the bloodstream for over 24 hours, so the purity of the product is crucial. A good guide is to check that the label shows the common name as well

Base cream recipe

(makes about 500 g, or 17¹/₂ oz)
200 ml (¹/₃ pt) sweet almond oil
40 g (1¹/₂ oz) beeswax granules or grated wax
Teaspoon wheatgerm oil

Put the beeswax in a toughened bowl. Pour in the almond oil and wheatgerm oil. Place the bowl in a pan of water over a gentle heat, to enable the wax to melt, stirring continuously to mix the ingredients. Take from the heat and keep stirring as the mixture cools. If you wish, you can add 10 drops of a favourite essential oil or a combination of up to three oils to make up 10 drops. When cool, dispense into suitable clean jars with screw lids. Store in a cool, dark place. The cream will keep for up to six months.

CAUTION: *If you are allergic to wheat do not add the wheatgerm oil, which is used as a preservative. This will not affect the quality of the cream, but will shorten its shelf-life and it will degenerate within three months.*

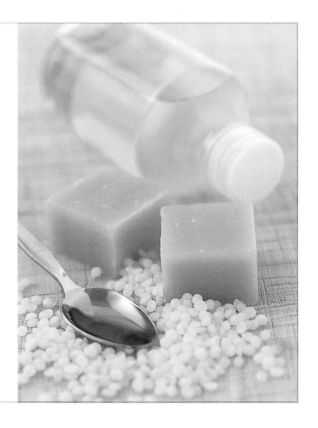

as the botanical Latin name and has specific instructions for use, including safety warnings. See that it is labelled "essential oil", which ensures that it contains 100 per cent concentrated plant oil, and look for a batch number, expiry date and the name and address of the supplier.

Avoid oils that are not correctly labelled – the more information, the better. Oils that are all one price are not usually pure; each essential oil should be individually priced. Essential oils should be sold in dark, glass bottles with a screw cap and stored away from direct light and heat. At home, store your oils in their dark glass bottles in a locked medicine cupboard well out of reach of children or pets. Keep the lid firmly closed, as the oils evaporate when exposed to the air. Most essential oils recommended for home use last for at least two years, depending on the oil and how often it is used.

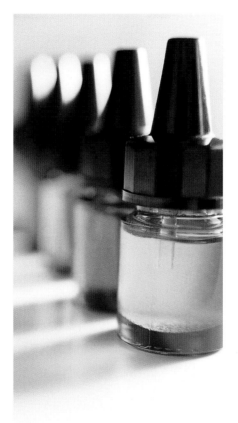

Blending oils and creams

Essential oils are highly potent and can be toxic if misused. When blending them with a carrier oil or cream, the motto is "less is best". It may be tempting to add an extra drop of essential oil but this may lead to a harmful reaction such as skin irritation. As you gain knowledge and experience from using pure essential oils, you may wish to create your own blends using a selection of different oils – but always follow the instructions and adhere strictly to the safety precautions.

To make an aromatic massage oil or cream, first wash your hands and check all utensils are clean and dry. Measure the required amount of carrier oil (a single oil or mixture of oils to make up the same quantity) or base cream into a suitable bowl, bottle or container. Now add your chosen pure essential oil. Mix with the cream or carrier oil by stirring with a cocktail stick or clean teaspoon. Wash your hands. Initially, it is best to err on the side of caution and use one drop of single pure essential oil to 10 ml (two teaspoons) of vegetable oil or 50 g (about 2 oz) of cream.

If you have sensitive skin, some essential oils such as black pepper, peppermint and Roman camomile, should be used sparingly – add one drop to 30 ml (six teaspoons) of oil or 150 g (about 5 oz) of cream. To help with measuring the base oil, you may prefer to use a 5 ml medicine spoon as teaspoons vary greatly in size. Buy essential oils in bottles with some form of built-in dropper that allows you to

note

To allow essential oils to be fully absorbed into the skin, do not wash hands or feet for at least an hour after they have been massaged.

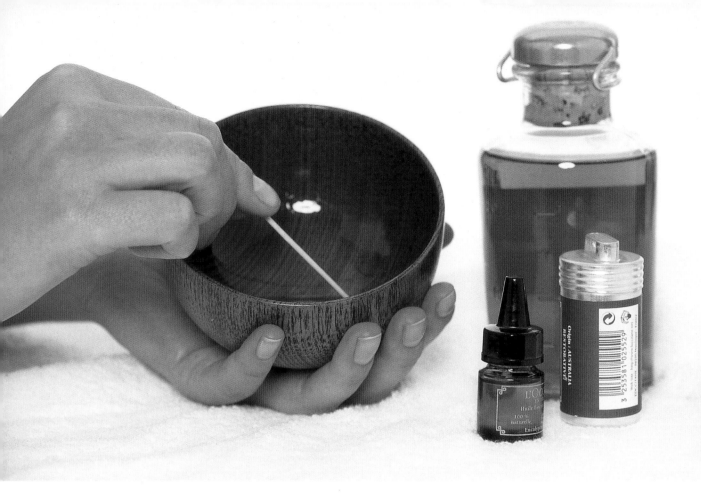

dispense one drop at a time with accuracy. If you accidentally add too much, mix in the appropriate amount of extra carrier oil or cream to restore the balance.

Remember, essential oils are very concentrated. If you wish to make up a larger quantity of massage oil or cream, work out the ratio of essential oil to carrier oil or cream – for example, you should add five drops of pure essential oil (two drops of Roman camomile, black pepper or peppermint) to 50 ml (10 teaspoons) of vegetable oil or 250 g (about 9 oz) of cream base. Once blended, ensure the lid is firmly in place, and label the bottle or pot clearly with date and ingredients. Keep in the fridge and use within one week.

Applying oil and cream

You need sufficient oil or cream to allow your hands to slip over the skin in a smooth and comfortable way, but not so much that your hands slide and you are unable to feel the underlying tissues. The amount needed obviously varies with each person depending on their skin type – and the size of their hands or feet! With practice and experience you will soon be able to judge correctly. Initially, it is best to opt for too little rather than too much. For hands, start with enough lubricant to cover a 5p piece and then top it up if necessary. (As feet are larger, use enough to cover a 10p piece.) Keep one hand in contact with the skin at all times, even when applying more lubricant, as withdrawing both hands can make your massage partner feel abandoned and vulnerable.

Oil or cream is best applied warm. Skin temperature, or a little warmer, is ideal. This provides a far more pleasant sensation for your partner and also encourages the absorption of the natural healing chemicals, so they can have a beneficial effect on mind and body. First wash your hands, then warm them, either by rubbing them briskly together or immersing them in a bowl of warm water for a few minutes. Now, place the oil or cream in the palm of one of your hands. Rub your hands together so they are well covered with lubricant and feel warm to touch. Do not apply lubricant directly to your partner's skin as this is not a very pleasant sensation.

Oil can be applied using a plastic bottle with an easy-to-use dispenser that prevents it pouring too quickly. Alternatively, place in a small plastic bowl. You can then dip in one or two fingers if you need more lubrication. If there is any oil left in the bowl at the end of the massage, throw it away immediately. Do not use again, as there is a risk of spreading infection. It is wise to place the bottle or bowl on a paper towel to absorb any oil spillage.

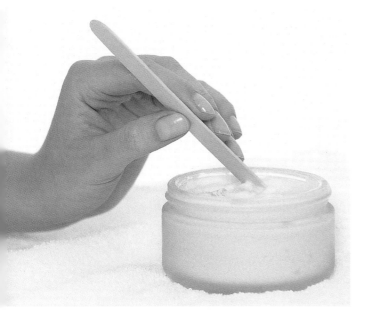

Cream should be taken from the pot and applied to your hands using a wooden or plastic spatula. This is for hygiene purposes, to prevent the spread of infection, and also for practical reasons as it means you can take the right amount. Take a tip from the beauty profession and place an extra blob on the top of one hand so you can replenish the cream without interrupting the massage. Always replace the lid on the cream pot or jar when not in use.

Sensitivity test

Some essential oils can cause skin reactions. So it is advisable to perform a patch test to check for sensitivity. Mix one drop of your chosen oil in a teaspoon of vegetable carrier oil. Rub a little of the blended oil on the inside of the wrist or behind the ears. Leave uncovered for 24 hours. Do not wash this area. Reactions often occur within a few hours. If you notice any signs of a rash, reddening or itchiness then do not use the oil. Rinse off immediately with cold water.

Using essential oils safely

- Always obtain oils from a reputable source, make sure they are clearly labelled and follow the instructions for use carefully. Dilute with carrier oil or base cream in the correct proportions.
- Use only the oils recommended for home use. Or ask a qualified, clinical aromatherapist for details of other suitable essential oils, and appropriate dilutions.
- Never apply to the skin neat (except lavender and tea tree) – always dilute with a carrier oil or base cream. Remove any accidental spills by gently scrubbing with a strong solution of washing up liquid.
- Be careful not to rub your eyes or lips when you have essential oil on your fingers (even diluted). If oil gets into eyes, rinse with sweet almond oil to ease the stinging. If in doubt, seek medical assistance.
- Do not take internally. If oils are consumed accidentally, get immediate medical help.
- Keep bottles out of reach of children and pets.
- Avoid using pure essential oils during pregnancy, when breastfeeding or on babies and children, unless advised by a fully qualified aromatherapist.
- Some oils can cause irritation and aggravate symptoms

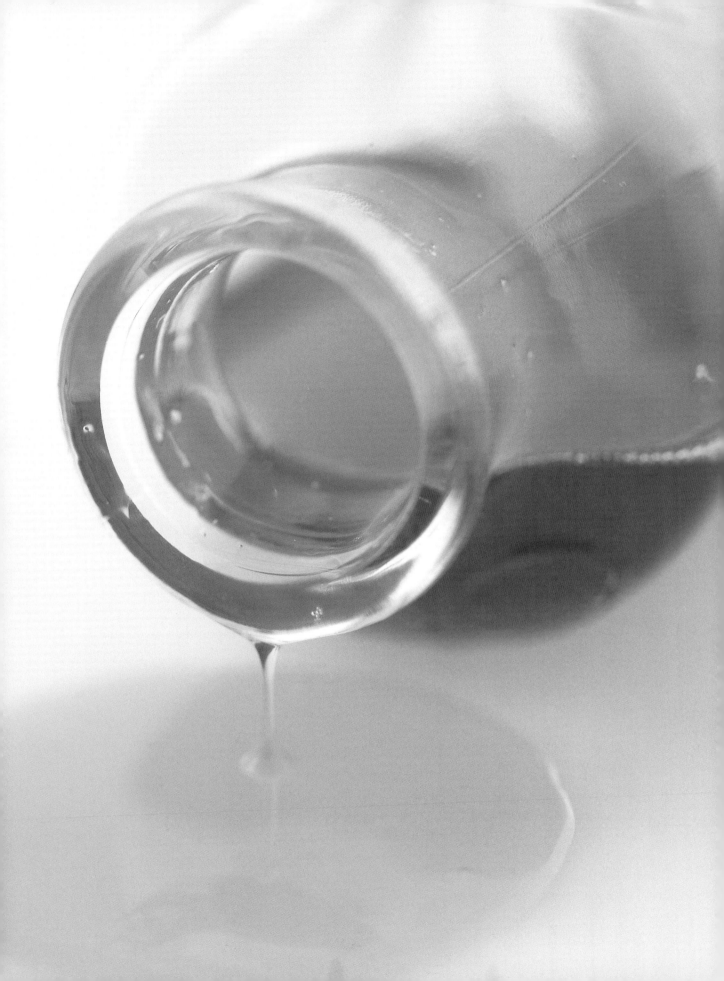

of certain medical conditions such as epilepsy, high blood pressure, asthma, hay fever and allergies. Check safety warnings and avoid problem oils. Always carry out a skin test (see page 29) to check for sensitivity.

- Seek professional advice if homeopathic medicines are being taken. Some essential oils may counteract the beneficial effects of the treatment.
- Do not use perfume or diffuse essential oils into the atmosphere while using essential oils for massage.
- It is not advisable to use one pure essential oil continually – whether you are giving or receiving the massage – as you can build up an intolerance or an accumulated toxic effect. Try alternating and varying the different oils for best effect.

Offer a choice

Let your massage partner choose a favourite aroma from a selection of pure essential oils. If you or your partner strongly dislike a particular fragrance, do not use it. If possible, smell a few different, essential oils before you buy. Some stores have test strips.

The origins of aromatherapy

Aromatherapy is the skilful application of essential oils in order to create a beneficial effect on mind and body. The word "aromatherapy", which literally means "curative treatment by the use of scent" was coined by the French cosmetic chemist Prof René Gattefosse, who studied the therapeutic powers of essential oils in the 1930s. His interest began when he accidentally burned his hand while carrying out an experiment in his laboratory. He plunged his hand into the nearest bowl of liquid, which happened to be pure lavender oil, and the pain eased immediately. His hand healed quickly with minimal scarring and there was no sign of infection.

Traditional beeswax

Beeswax is an ancient ingredient in moisturizing creams. As long ago as AD150, the Greek physician Galen created a cold cream that was a mixture of melted beeswax and olive oil, with the addition of water or scented water. The recipe has been refined over the years but beeswax remains an important ingredient for anyone wishing to create their own massage creams. Beeswax thickens vegetable oils to a suitable consistency for massage, and also has healing properties of its own. It keeps the skin in good condition and can be helpful in treating minor skin disorders. Natural, unbleached, yellow beeswax is preferable to bleached, white beeswax, as it is more likely to be free from chemicals. Beeswax is available in most health food stores and can be grated or used in granular form to make base creams to which pure essential oils can be added.

Recommended carrier oils

There is a wide choice of base or carrier oils. Here is a selection of the oils most suitable for hand and foot massage.

Apricot kernel (Prunus armenaica)

This oil is extracted from the seed kernels of the apricot tree. It is pale yellow and has many similarities to sweet almond oil. It is a good source of minerals and vitamins, especially vitamin A, and is readily absorbed into the skin.

USE: Apricot kernel oil is rich, nourishing and soothing, making it beneficial for dry, ageing and sensitive skin. It can be used on its own as a light massage oil, or mixed with another vegetable oil, such as sweet almond oil. Apricot kernel oil combines well with all pure essential oils recommended for home use. A useful alternative is peach kernel (Prunus persica) which shares many of the same properties.

CAUTIONS: Generally well tolerated.

Borage seed *(Borago officinalis)*

This oil comes from the seeds of the borage plant. Pale yellow, it is an excellent source of vitamins, minerals and essential fatty acids, especially gamma linolenic acid (GLA).

USE: Borage seed oil has valuable moisturizing properties and is suitable for all skin types. It is reputed to be an anti-ageing rejuvenator for more mature skins, and can help to soothe skin conditions such as eczema and psoriasis. However, it is a very sticky oil so it is not suitable for massage on its own. Blend in a 1:9 dilution with a lighter-textured carrier oil, such as sweet almond oil, and use as a massage oil or when making a cream base. Add pure essential oils as appropriate.

CAUTIONS: Generally well tolerated.

Evening primrose *(Oenothera biennis)*

Evening primrose oil, which is golden yellow, is derived from the seeds of the plant. It is rich in essential fatty acids, especially gamma linolenic acid (GLA), and is probably best known as a nutritional supplement to treat menstrual and pre-menstrual problems. However, evening primrose oil can also be applied to the skin through massage to provide additional therapeutic benefits.

USE: Evening primrose oil is a good skin softener and moisturizer and particularly useful for dry, ageing or chapped skin. Due to the high GLA content, it can also be helpful for soothing skin conditions such as eczema and psoriasis. Evening primrose oil is quite sticky so it is best added to a lighter, more freely flowing carrier oil such as sweet almond oil in a 1:9 dilution. This blend can be used as a massage oil or when making a cream base. Pure essential oils can be added, if you wish.

CAUTIONS: Generally well tolerated. Store away from light and heat.

Jojoba *(Simmondsia chinensis)*

Jojoba (pronounced ho-ho-ba) oil comes from the fruit of an evergreen desert plant. Although referred to as an oil, it is actually a liquid wax that is semi-solid at room temperature and solidifies when refrigerated. It is light yellow, almost odourless and readily absorbed by the skin. Jojoba oil has a similar chemical structure to sebum, the skin's own natural cleanser and moisturizer, and contains protein, minerals and vitamin E, a natural antioxidant (and so has anti-ageing properties).

USE: Jojoba oil is a very useful carrier oil for massage as it is suitable for all skin types, including irritated conditions, and has an excellent moisturizing and nourishing effect. However, jojoba oil is very expensive so it is best used in small quantities – dilute in a ratio of 1:9 with another carrier oil such as sweet almond oil.

CAUTIONS: Generally well tolerated.

Sweet almond *(Prunus amygdalus)*

This is extracted from the kernels of the sweet almond tree. It is pale yellow and slightly viscous, with a mild, nutty fragrance. Rich in minerals, vitamins and protein, sweet almond oil is widely available, highly versatile and has a longer shelf-life than many other vegetable oils.

USES: Sweet almond oil is one of the most popular carrier oils for hand and foot massage because it is both light and smooth to use. It is ideal for beginners as it can be used on its own, or mixed with other carrier oils and with pure essential oils recommended for home use. It is also a useful ingredient in home-made massage creams. Sweet almond oil helps soften and nourish the skin, and is especially beneficial for dry, sensitive and irritated skin conditions.

CAUTIONS: Generally well tolerated. Do not confuse sweet almond oil with the oil made from bitter almonds, which has culinary applications but is never used in massage.

Wheatgerm *(Triticum vulgare)*

Wheatgerm oil is deep orange-brown with a strong, earthy fragrance. It has a high nutrient content – it is one of the best sources of vitamin E, a natural antioxidant (and so has anti-ageing properties) – and is rich in other vitamins, proteins and minerals.

USE: Wheatgerm oil is recognized as being beneficial in repairing scar tissue and soothing burns. It is also useful for revitalizing ageing and dry skins, and can help relieve tired muscles. As wheatgerm oil is so rich and viscous it is rarely used on its own. Blend with other carrier oils in a 1:9 dilution. Due to its antioxidant properties, wheatgerm helps prolong the shelf-life of less stable oils by a month or so.

CAUTIONS: May not be tolerated well by some people. Do not use on people with a wheat allergy.

Recommended essential oils

These oils are safe to use at home so long as you dilute them with a suitable carrier oil or base cream in the correct proportions. Follow safety warnings.

Black Pepper *(Piper nigrum)*

This pale olive, warm, spice-scented oil is extracted from dried, crushed black peppercorns, which are the fruit of a woody vine that is native to eastern Asia. For many centuries, black pepper has been highly regarded as a culinary and medicinal spice both in the Far East and Europe. It is reputed that Attila the Hun demanded large quantities of black pepper as part of the ransom for the city of Rome.

USE: Black pepper has a warming, stimulating effect that makes it a useful ingredient in an oil or cream for massaging hands and feet. It is commonly added to massage blends to relax tired muscles and help alleviate muscular pain and stiffness. It can also be used to loosen stiff joints and aid mobility. And, as it helps boost blood circulation, it is a good oil to choose for people with circulatory problems – it can be particularly beneficial for unbroken chilblains. On an emotional level, black pepper is mentally invigorating and is often used to encourage a "fighting spirit".

CAUTIONS: Generally well tolerated but may be an irritant in some people because of its skin warming properties. If you have sensitive skin, use very sparingly – one drop to 30 ml (six teaspoons) of carrier oil or 150g (about 5 oz) of cream. Test before using by applying a little diluted oil to the skin and waiting for any reaction. Do not use with homeopathic remedies (and store far away from them), as it may counteract their benefits. Seek the advice of a qualified clinical aromatherapist for use in pregnancy, when breastfeeding, or for babies and children.

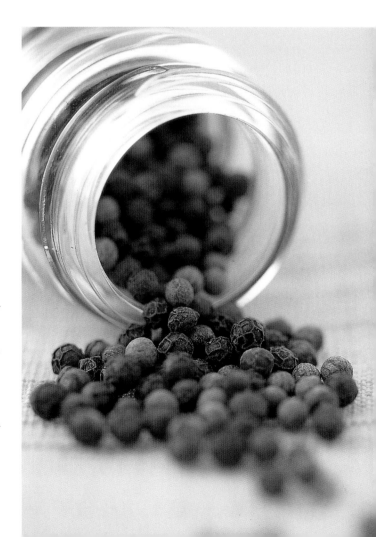

Cedarwood *(Cedrus atlanticus)*

This yellowish oil is extracted from the aromatic wood of the evergreen tree, the atlas cedar. Cedarwood is thought to be one of the first recognized essential oils and is still used today in traditional Tibetan medicine. It has a mild, woody fragrance that can be more appealing to men than the floral scents of other essential oils.

USE: Cedarwood has astringent and antiseptic properties, making it useful for a range of skin complaints, especially itchy conditions or fungal infections. It is a warm, stimulating oil that acts as a tonic to the whole body and can be helpful for improving poor circulation and relieving the pain of arthritis and rheumatism. The effect on the nervous system is sedative, helping to ease tension and boost confidence. Cedarwood is also regarded as an aphrodisiac, so it makes a good choice for a sensual massage.

CAUTIONS: Do not use during pregnancy, when breastfeeding, or on babies or young children. It may cause irritation on some skins, so test before using by applying a little diluted oil to the skin and waiting for any reaction. Check the botanical name on the label before buying, as there are several varieties.

Frankincense *(Boswellia carteri)*

This pale yellow or greenish oil, which is extracted from the small tree's natural gum resin, has a warm, rich, sweet, woody odour. Frankincense was one of the three gifts presented to baby Jesus by the three Wise Kings as a sign of reverence. It was so highly prized at the time that it was almost as precious as gold.

USE: Frankincense is suitable for all skin types, but is particularly useful for moisturizing and gently soothing dry and mature skin. This essential oil is added to massage creams and oils to aid relaxation and alleviate mental and physical lethargy. It is known for its ability to induce deep, slow breathing and is often used during meditation to promote concentrated and focused thought. Frankincense is often favoured by men.

CAUTIONS: Generally well tolerated. Seek the advice of a qualified clinical aromatherapist for use in pregnancy, when breastfeeding, or for babies and children.

Geranium *(Pelargonium graveolens)*

This pale-green oil is extracted from the leaves of the popular window-box plant, traditionally grown to keep evil spirits away. It is a highly versatile oil and popular for massage. The refreshing rose-like floral scent is best appreciated when diluted in a carrier oil or base cream.

USE: Geranium has a balancing effect on the sebaceous glands, so making it useful for all skin types, especially very dry or very oily skin. Geranium oil is reputed to stimulate the circulation of blood around the body and boost the lymphatic system for speedy disposal of toxins and excess fluids. Mix with a carrier oil to massage the hands and feet of anyone suffering from poor circulation and stiff joints. It is also an uplifting tonic for low moods and helps calm an over-active mind.

CAUTIONS: May irritate very sensitive skin. Test before using by applying a little diluted oil to the skin and waiting for a reaction. Seek the advice of a qualified clinical aromatherapist for use in pregnancy, when breastfeeding, or for babies and children.

Lavender *(Lavendula angustifolio)*

The oil is extracted from the fresh, flowering tops of the plant. It is clear or faintly yellow with a light, fresh, floral aroma. The name derives from the Latin word "lavare", which means "to wash". In Tudor times, women scattered lavender over their floors to cleanse and deodorize the rooms.

USE: Lavender is a good oil to choose when you are new to using pure essential oils. Indeed, it is so versatile that it may be the only one you need! Combine with sweet almond oil for an excellent all-purpose massage oil that can be used on most people on most occasions. Lavender is a conditioner for all skin types and aids the healing

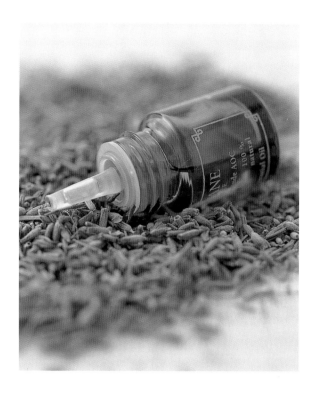

to China. The fruit was a traditional gift offered to the mandarins of China, hence the name.

USE: Mandarin is useful when massaging elderly or frail people as it works in a very gentle but effective way to balance the mind and body. It can act as a mildly stimulating tonic, helping to boost circulation and lymphatic drainage, and also as a gentle sedative for reducing stress and tension. The fruity aroma brings a sense of cheerfulness, which can ease loneliness and uplift low spirits. It is suitable for all skin types and is commonly used in skin care preparations for cleansing oily skin and for aiding the healing process and helping to prevent scarring.

CAUTIONS: Generally well tolerated but may be slightly phototoxic (sensitizes the skin to the sun's rays). Wait at least an hour after a massage before exposing the skin to strong sunlight or ultra violet rays. Considered safe and beneficial during pregnancy when added to a base oil to massage aching hands and feet. However, always seek the advice of a qualified clinical aromatherapist for use in pregnancy, when breastfeeding, or for babies and children.

process of skin conditions. It has painkilling qualities that make it useful for conditions such as arthritis. Lavender is so mild that it can be used directly on the skin (but check with a qualified aromatherapist first), and also acts as an antiseptic, so it can be used to treat burns, stings and bites. A natural sedative, it is often used to alleviate insomnia and aid restful sleep. Lavender helps induce feelings of peace, contentment and tranquillity.

CAUTIONS: Generally well tolerated, although some people do not like the smell. Do not use in the first three months of pregnancy. Can be useful in labour and for young children but always seek the advice of a qualified clinical aromatherapist for use in pregnancy, when breastfeeding, or for babies and children.

Mandarin *(Citrus reticulata)*

This mild yet energizing oil is golden-yellow with a delicate, mood-enhancing citrus scent. It is extracted from the rind of the fruit of the mandarin tree, which is native

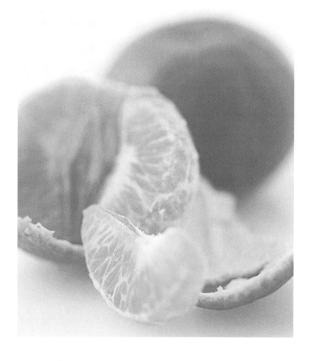

Peppermint *(Mentha piperata)*

This mint-scented oil is extracted from the same flowering herb that grows in many gardens in the UK. Pale yellow or greenish in colour, it is traditionally associated with brightness and cleanliness.

USE: Soothing and cooling, peppermint oil is a popular ingredient in massage oils and creams for refreshing and revitalizing sore, overworked feet. It is useful for easing muscular aches and pains and lifting fatigue. The strong, fresh fragrance of peppermint oil can help overcome tiredness and induce clarity of thought when the mind is confused.

CAUTIONS: Use very sparingly – one drop to 30ml (six teaspoons) of carrier oil or 150g (about 5 oz) of cream. Can cause slight irritation on sensitive skins. Test before using by applying a little diluted oil to the skin and waiting for any reaction. Do not use with homeopathic remedies (and store far away from them), as it may counteract their benefits. Do not use in the evening – it may disturb sleep. Avoid using too frequently. Not to be used during pregnancy, when breastfeeding, or for babies and children.

Roman camomile *(Anthemis nobilis)*

This pale yellow oil has a mild, sweet slightly fruity aroma. It is extracted from the daisy-like white flower heads of the perennial herb. Camomile has long been recognized for its medicinal and cosmetic properties. The ancient Egyptians held it in such high regard that the plant was declared sacred and dedicated to Ra, the sun god.

USE: When appropriately used, Roman camomile is a gentle, soothing oil that is useful for dry, red and sensitive skin. It is often applied to treat itchy skin conditions, especially those associated with emotional stress. Very effective in mixing with oils and creams to massage dull muscular aches, it is also useful for relieving the pain and inflammation of joint conditions such as arthritis. Roman camomile has a calming effect on the mind and body and is beneficial for all stress-related disorders. Use at the end of a long, tiring day to lift anxieties, doubts and worries.

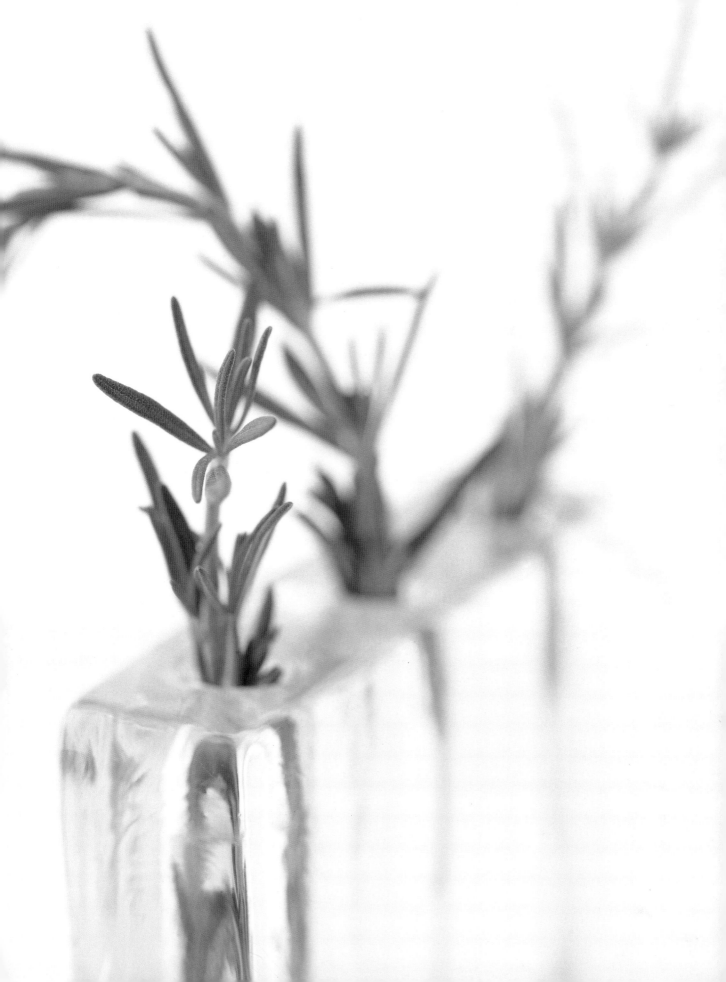

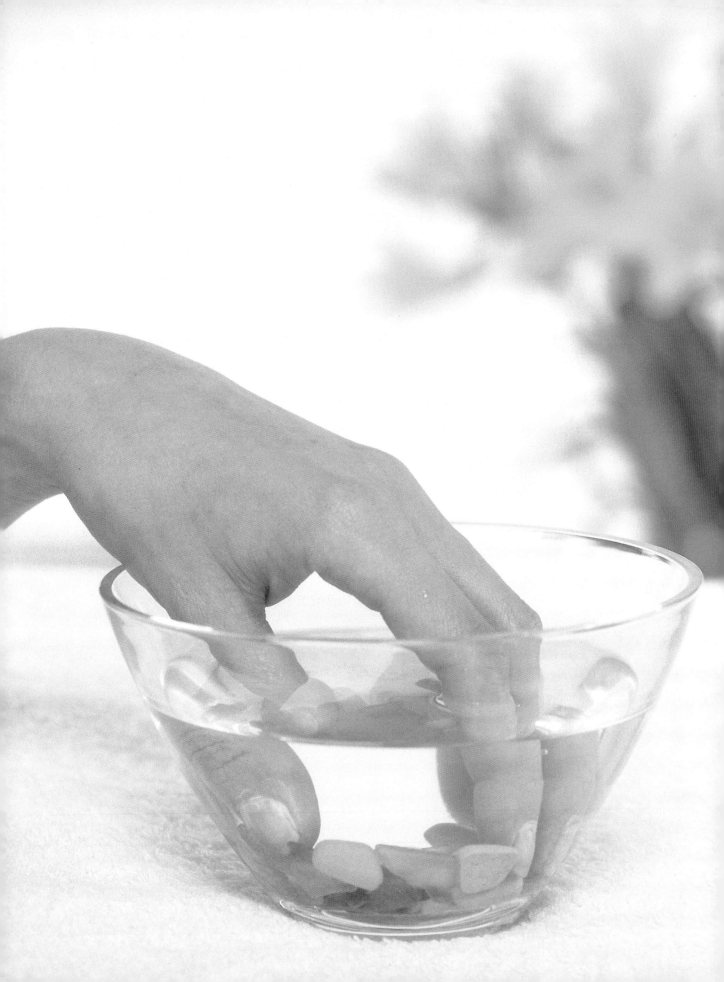

CAUTIONS: Use very sparingly – one drop to 30 ml (six teaspoons) of carrier oil or 150g (about 5 oz) of cream. It may cause irritation on sensitive skins. Test before using by applying a little diluted oil to the skin and waiting for any reaction. Can be a beneficial oil for adding to a massage blend to calm irritable or anxious children, but always seek the advice of a qualified clinical aromatherapist for use in pregnancy, when breastfeeding, or for babies and children.

Rosemary *(Rosmarinus officinalis)*

This clear or pale-yellow oil is extracted from the fresh flowering tips or leaves of the evergreen bush and has a strong, woody scent. The herb has long been associated with lifting mental fatigue and improving alertness. The ancient Greeks put twigs of rosemary in their hair to boost their concentration during examinations. Ophelia in Shakespeare's Hamlet refers to its memory-enhancing powers when she says: "There's rosemary, that's for remembrance."

USE: Rosemary can be helpful in easing aches and pains. Add to your massage oil or cream for people with arthritis, rheumatism and tired, overworked hands and feet. It is an invigorating, energizing oil that strengthens the mind and stimulates blood circulation – so it is useful for massaging unbroken chilblains. Rosemary is suitable for all skin types and has long been used in skin care – it is an ingredient of true eau de cologne.

CAUTIONS: May irritate sensitive skin. Test before using by applying a little diluted oil to the skin and waiting for any reaction. Do not use if the person suffers from epilepsy or high blood pressure. Not to be used during pregnancy, when breastfeeding, or for babies and children.

Tea tree *(Melaleuca alternifolia)*

Not to be confused with the traditional British beverage, tea tree oil is extracted from the leaves and twigs of a small tree or shrub belonging to the same family as the powerfully scented eucalyptus. It is a pale yellow-greenish oil with a strong medicinal smell that acts quickly and effectively to alleviate a wide range of conditions. Indeed, it is one of only a few essential oils that have undergone extensive clinical studies into its therapeutic qualities.

USE: Tea tree oil is best known for its anti-infection properties and has been shown to be active against bacteria, fungi and viruses. It is a stimulating, energizing oil and helps boost the immune system so that it responds to infection more effectively. It was included in tropical first aid kits during the Second World War to help fight disease. Tea tree is so mild that it can be used directly on the skin (but check with a qualified aromatherapist first), and is useful in treating athlete's foot, verrucae, warts, blisters, cuts and bites. It is also beneficial for soothing aching feet or wrists. If you are sensitive to tea tree oil, an alternative is Niaouli (Melaleuca viridiflora), which is a member of the same plant family and has similar properties.

CAUTIONS: Generally well tolerated but some people may be sensitive. Test before using by applying a little diluted oil to the skin and waiting for any reaction. Seek the advice of a qualified clinical aromatherapist for use in pregnancy, when breastfeeding, or for babies and children.

Pamper your feet

Bathe your hands or feet in a bowl half full of warm water. Add three drops of a suitable essential oil: peppermint to revitalize, lavender to relax, geranium to boost circulation or tea tree to deodorize and fight fungal infection. Soak hands or feet for around five minutes – no longer or you will start to upset the balance of natural protective oils on the skin. Enjoy the benefits!

Massage is a basic, nurturing instinct. Massage has also been described as one of the oldest forms of healing.

Preparing
4
for massage

Since ancient times, people all over the world have used the natural therapeutic power of touch in their everyday lives. Once you have learnt a few simple techniques, you can use your natural skills to give a safe and effective hand or foot massage to family and friends.

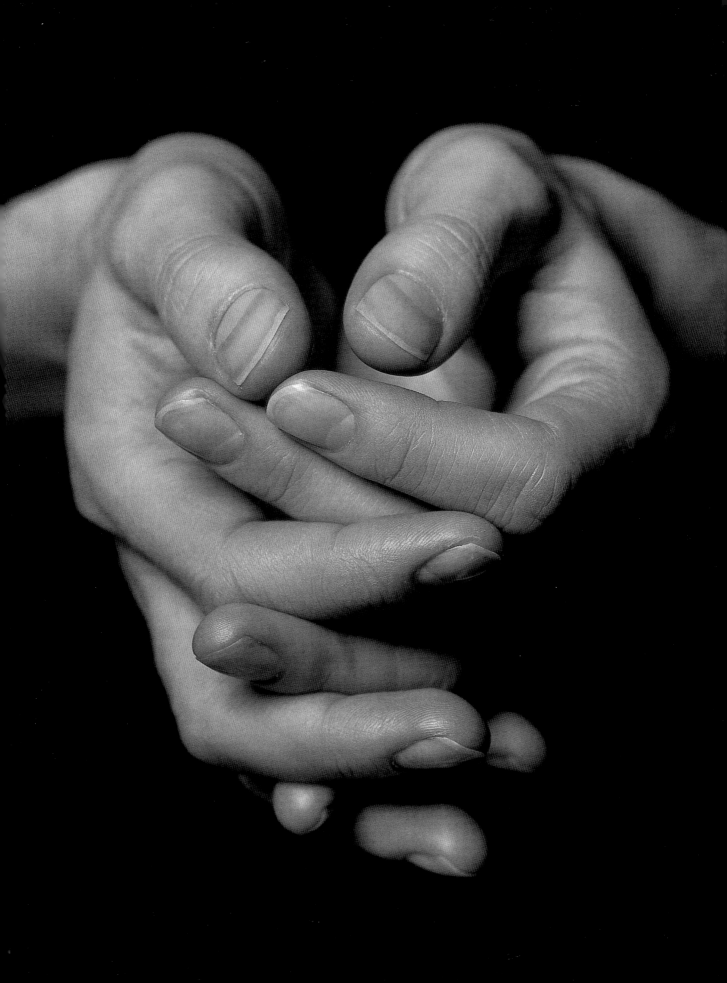

Hand and foot massage techniques

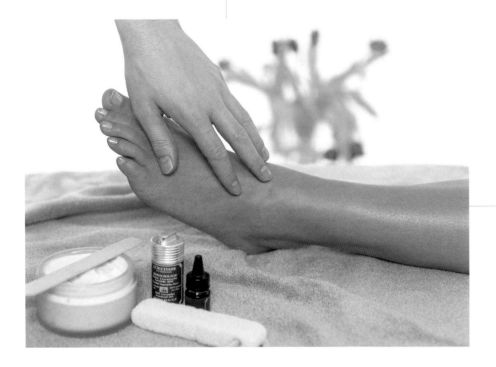

Massage of any kind can be classified as the manipulation of the body's soft tissues – the skin, fat, muscle and connective tissue such as tendons and ligaments. It involves a series of movements using your hands. Each movement is applied in a particular way with the aim of having a specific therapeutic effect on the area being massaged.

As Hippocrates wrote in around 460–375BC, "rubbing can bind a joint that it is too loose and also loosen a joint that is too hard". Massage can be stimulating or sedating. It can be performed gently or vigorously. So, it is necessary to know the effects and benefits of different "rubbing" or massaging movements before you begin. The main movements used in hand and foot massage are: stroking, effleurage, kneading and tapping.

Stroking

Your hands and feet are well supplied with sensory nerve endings that respond to touch by sending signals to the brain and influencing the way you feel, both mentally and physically. The powerful impact of stroking shows that touch does not have to be deep to be beneficial. Soft stroking helps soothe and calm the sensory nerves, sending waves of pleasure throughout the body. It has an almost soporific effect and can be used at any time during the massage to help relax and reassure your partner. Faster, more energetic stroking is energizing and revitalizing, and a great way of pepping up the circulation to warm your extremities in chilly weather.

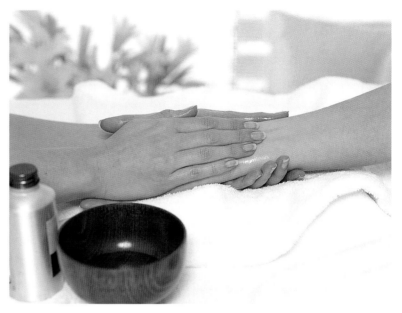

A hand or foot massage begins with gentle stroking to spread the oil or cream, and familiarize both giver and receiver with the sensation of skin to skin contact. It is used to calm and relax between more vigorous movements, and again at the end of the massage to bring it to a relaxing conclusion. Gentle stroking is a slow, light and superficial gliding movement, your hands and fingers are supple and slightly cupped so they mould naturally to the bends and curves of the part being massaged. It is a smooth, rhythmical and repetitive action that is beneficial for both giver and receiver. Indeed, studies show that stroking a pet is an effective way of reducing stress levels and improving general well-being – and giving a massage can be an equally rewarding experience.

Feathering is a form of gentle stroking that has an almost instant calming effect on the sensory nerve endings. Feathering can be used at any time between movements and is often used as a final stroke to conclude the massage. It is particularly beneficial when massaging someone who is elderly, frail or anxious, and it is effective with babies, too. Use the tips of your fingers to stroke the skin very lightly and softly as though massaging it with a feather. Release your touch very, very slowly at the end of each stroke so that your hands float smoothly away.

Effleurage

This movement is the basis of any massage. The name is derived from the French word "effleurer", which means "to skim over". It is a similar movement to stroking but is generally a firmer, smoothing action. Slow effleurage with a light or moderate pressure flows on naturally from gentle stroking and helps prepare the area for subsequent deeper massage movements. Once the soft tissues start to relax, you may choose to use more energizing strokes with a faster action and deeper pressure. Effleurage is a useful linking movement between different strokes. And, if you are unsure what to do next, try a few effleurage strokes. You can give a pleasurable massage by using effleurage strokes alone.

Effleurage strokes are usually directed towards the heart, so helping to boost the flow of deoxygenated blood through the veins, and of lymph taking impurities back to the heart. The venous and lymphatic systems are mainly driven by the movement of the muscles, and so tend to become sluggish, especially as we get older and less active. Your pressure should be firmer on the upward stroke toward the body, using a light touch on the return movements. Use the flat of your hands or fleshy pads of your finger, or thumbs, as appropriate. Keep your wrists flexible and your hands supple and flowing in a long continuous sequence. Maintain contact with your partner at all times.

Kneading

This is a deeper movement than effleurage so it is mainly used on fleshier areas. Your hands do not glide over the surface of the skin but press much deeper so you can feel the skin moving against the soft tissues beneath to detect and relax specific areas of tension.

The action is similar to kneading dough. Your hands should be relaxed and supple as you pick up the soft tis-

note

Do not worry about feeling awkward at first. Instead of trying to get every stroke technically correct, concentrate on massaging with care and affection to make your partner feel relaxed, nurtured and secure. With practice, your massage will flow freely and smoothly.

tip

Practise the different movements on yourself to feel the effect of varying the speed or pressure of the strokes.

sues, separate them from the underlying structures, compress them and then allow them to relax. The movement is slow and rhythmic with a deep but comfortable pressure. The fleshy pads of your fingers or thumbs move in a circular motion with an increase in pressure on the upward half of the circle and a decrease on the downward half. Once the circle is complete, your hand moves smoothly to the next part so that contact and rhythm are maintained. Be careful not to pinch or work too long in one area as this may cause discomfort.

Kneading is very effective in reducing the pain, tension and stiffness often felt in hands and feet. It is a wonderful releasing movement for taut muscles and aching joints, and has a positive effect on stimulating blood and lymph circulation. The rhythmical compression and relaxation of your hands acts like a pump to boost the flow of blood back to the heart and speed the flow of lymph to the nearest set of lymph nodes to be cleansed and filtered. However, as it creates so much heat, do not knead over arthritic, painful, hot or inflamed joints.

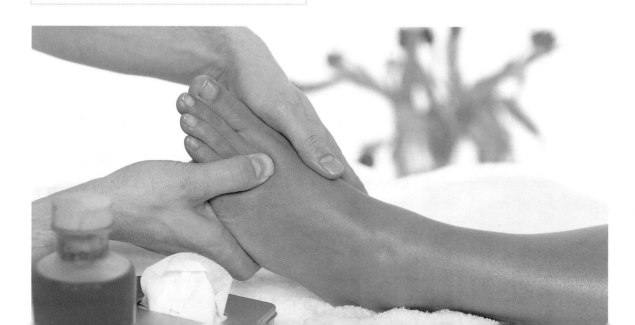

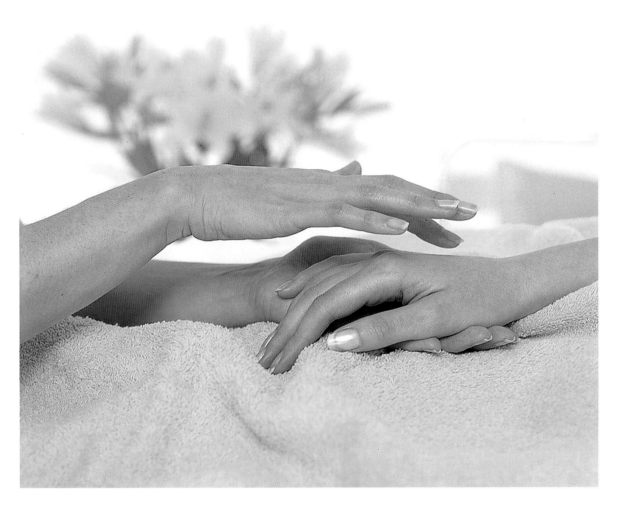

Tapping

This is an invigorating movement that strengthens slack muscles, warms the area and stimulates sensory nerve endings. It can play an important part in an energizing, circulation-boosting routine but should not be used when massaging babies, children, elderly, arthritic or frail people as it may be too vigorous. Tapping involves striking the skin and then releasing in the same rapid, rhythmical way as a percussion instrument in an orchestra. Keep your wrists flexible and use your hands or fingers to tap the skin with a light, springy movement. Your hands or fingers bounce back up as soon as they land on the skin. It is best to start and finish each tapping sequence with a lighter pressure to avoid an abrupt shock. Do not use tapping movements until the area has been warmed and prepared with stroking or effleurage movements. Use gentle strokes afterward to soothe the sensory nerve endings and aid the flow of any excess blood or lymph back to the heart.

tip

With any form of massage it is important to remember that you are working "with" and not "on" another person – hence the term "massage partner" used throughout this book.

Giving a safe massage

Hand and foot massage is generally considered to be a safe, non-invasive therapy that is suitable for most people. Indeed, it is often given in hospitals, hospices and nursing homes as it is so comforting for elderly, frail or ill people. However, it is important not to launch straight into action without being aware of the safety guidelines you should follow – before, during and after a massage – which ensure your partner enjoys the optimum benefits from a hand or foot massage.

When to massage with extra care

Massage is likely to bring many benefits to most people. However, before you begin your massage, it is essential to set time aside to discuss any relevant health issues or concerns. You need to know your massage partner's state of health so that you are prepared for any problems that may arise during the massage, and how to deal with them. You should also be aware that there are a few occasions when it is not advisable to give a hand or foot massage, or when it is important to show sensitivity and massage with great care. If a foot massage is not appropriate, then offer a hand massage, and vice versa.

- Seek advice from an appropriate medical practitioner if your massage partner has a chronic (on going) medical condition such as a serious heart problem, oedema (fluid retention leading to tissue swelling), epilepsy or diabetes.

- Do not give a foot massage if your partner has a recent history of thrombosis (blood clots in an artery or vein) or embolism (blockage in an artery). There is a slight chance that massage may encourage a clot to break away and enter the bloodstream. A light hand massage is appropriate and usually beneficial.

- Do not massage hands or feet that show signs of a contagious or infectious skin or nail condition such as fungal nail or athlete's foot (see Chapter Nine). Massage could irritate and/or spread it. There is also a slight risk that you may contract the disease. You can massage over very dry skin or rashes so long as the skin is not open and the condition is not contagious.

- Do not massage over new scar tissue or following recent surgery to the area as it may hinder the healing process.

- Avoid massaging directly over warts, moles, bruises, abrasions, open cuts, broken skin, blisters, bites, stings, unexplained lumps, bumps and areas of sunburn. Cover with a small plaster, if possible, and massage gently around the site to encourage the natural healing process. You should also cover any cuts or abrasions on your own hands to reduce the risk of cross infection.

- Treat protruding or varicose veins with care. Brush your hands lightly over veins without exerting any pressure.

- Do not massage directly over any injuries and sprains or fragile bones. Avoid inflamed, swollen or painful joints as massage creates heat that may aggravate the condition. Do not try to reshape malformed toes – massage around them.

note

If you have any doubts – do not give a massage. Trust your intuition and postpone the massage until you have taken professional advice or are certain the condition has cleared up completely.

- Massage is not usually recommended for anyone with a very high temperature. This generally indicates that the body is bringing its defence mechanisms into action to deal with an infection. Massage may interfere with the natural healing process – and there is also a risk that an infection may be passed on to you.

- Postpone your massage if you or your massage partner feel generally unwell or nauseous.

- Be cautious during pregnancy (see page 91), especially during the first three months. Keep strokes light and gentle (avoid massaging the abdomen). Do not use pure essential oils during pregnancy and breastfeeding with-out the advice of a qualified clinical aromatherapist.

- Take great care when massaging the feet of people with poor circulation and/or a history of leg ulcers. Massage can be beneficial but it is imperative not to damage or irritate the skin.

note

Your hands need to be well coordinated and flexible to perform the variety of massage movements effectively, so practise a few mobility exercises every day (see pages 116–19). Hard, tense hands cannot give a fluent massage and may even cause pain or discomfort.

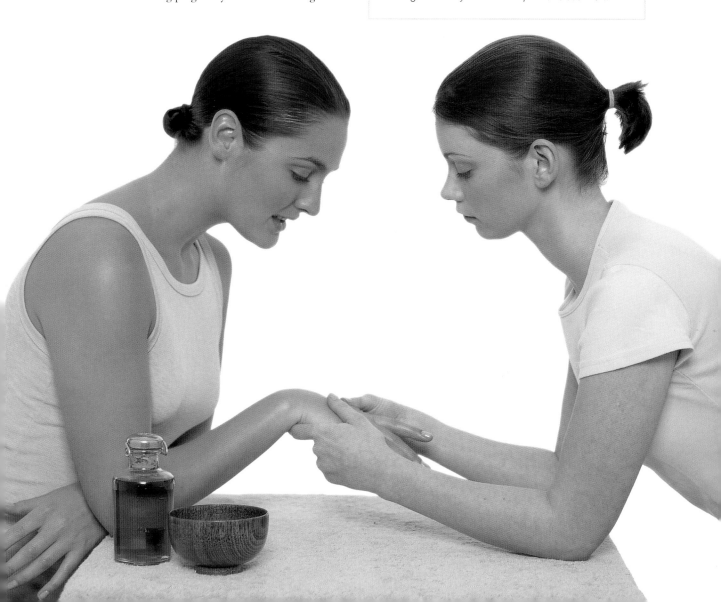

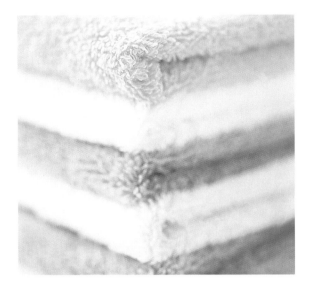

During massage

Your partner may experience a range of reactions during massage – which may take you both by surprise. So you should be prepared and know how to react.

- Some people find that a massage on hands and feet can tickle. If an area is ticklish, try giving a slower, firmer massage. It may be a sign that your massage partner is feeling a little uptight, insecure or nervous about the massage – which is quite understandable when trying something new. Ask him or her to take some deep breaths and try to let go of anxieties.
- People may feel very sleepy during the massage. This is a sign that their body needs sleep, so tell them not to fight it. Ensure that their head and body are well supported, and continue the massage as usual. Gently awaken them at the end of the massage and allow time for them to gather their thoughts.
- In some situations, receiving a soothing, caring massage can release emotional blockages and your massage partner may start to express fears, anxieties and sadness. Be prepared to pay attention without being seen to interfere or judge. All you can do is listen and express sympathy. Be sensitive to the mood and ask if your massage partner would like

you to continue or stop and talk. If you are massaging within a professional healthcare setting, it is advisable to learn more about listening skills.

- Some people suddenly feel hot and flushed or tingly as blood circulation is increased to the extremities. Others feel cold and shivery as their body temperature falls with their increasing sense of relaxation. Be aware of their body language and be prepared to meet their needs. Turn down the heat in the room or provide a blanket for warmth. If your massage partner feels light-headed or dizzy, offer a glass of water and suggest that they rest awhile before moving.
- Be aware of any tension creeping into your massage partner's hands or feet as you massage. Some people find it hard to relax, so you may need to give some gentle reminders to help them let go and enjoy the benefits. Just telling them to "relax" will not help – use gentle soothing massage strokes or suggest they take deep breaths. Many people respond well to visualizations, which are really just formalized daydreams. Suggest that your massage partner imagines that they are in a pleasant location that has positive associations – a beach or a pretty wooded glade, perhaps. Encourage your massage partner to spend a few minutes in this place using their senses to recreate a joyful feeling of "being there", both physically and mentally.
- Your depth of pressure may cause discomfort if it is too light or too deep. Always check with your massage partner – and be especially careful with older people and children. Massage should never cause pain. Ask your massage partner to tell you at once if any movement feels uncomfortable or unpleasant. You can easily stop and then continue with another movement. Take note of the recipient's body language – be aware of any twitches, winces or groans that could be a sign of discomfort.

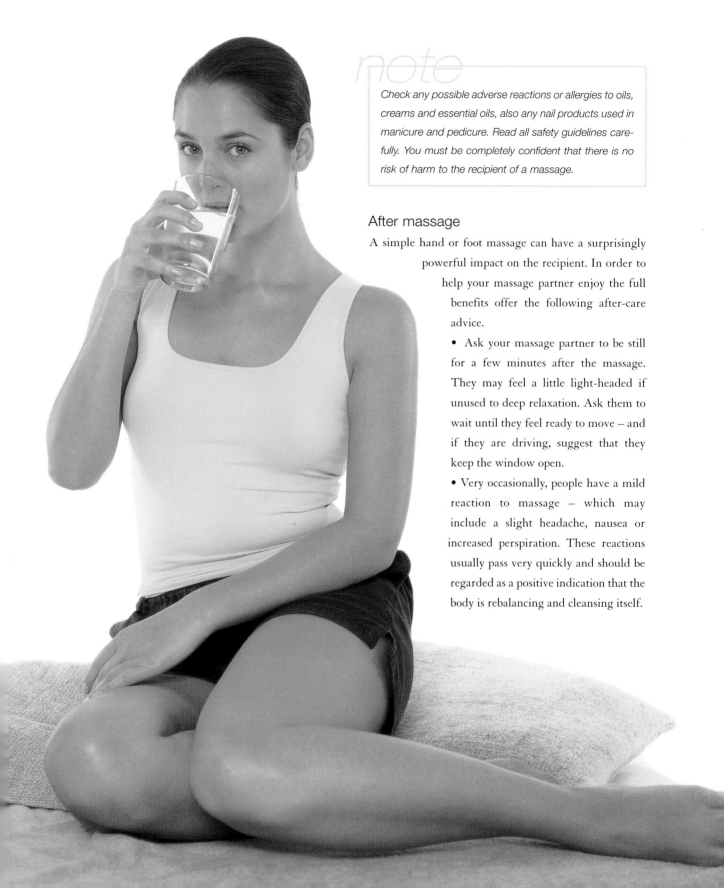

Check any possible adverse reactions or allergies to oils, creams and essential oils, also any nail products used in manicure and pedicure. Read all safety guidelines carefully. You must be completely confident that there is no risk of harm to the recipient of a massage.

After massage

A simple hand or foot massage can have a surprisingly powerful impact on the recipient. In order to help your massage partner enjoy the full benefits offer the following after-care advice.

• Ask your massage partner to be still for a few minutes after the massage. They may feel a little light-headed if unused to deep relaxation. Ask them to wait until they feel ready to move – and if they are driving, suggest that they keep the window open.

• Very occasionally, people have a mild reaction to massage – which may include a slight headache, nausea or increased perspiration. These reactions usually pass very quickly and should be regarded as a positive indication that the body is rebalancing and cleansing itself.

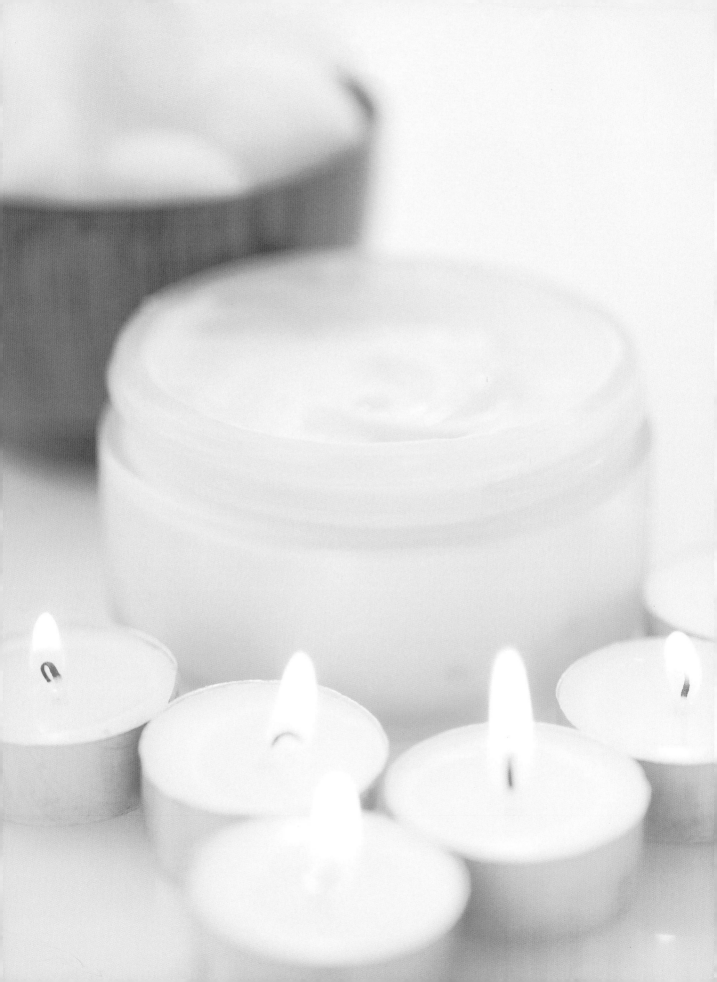

- Advise your massage partner to drink plenty of still water and herbal teas to speed up the elimination of toxins from the body. They should also cut back on tea, coffee and colas, which act like a diuretic (increasing the flow of urine out of the body) and should try to avoid smoking or drinking alcohol for at least twelve hours.

- Heavy meals should be avoided straight after (and immediately before) any form of massage. The demands of digestion will divert energy away from the natural healing process. Light snacks and fresh fruit are best.

tip

After giving a massage you need time to replenish your own energy. Avoid rushing on to the next job or giving another massage, set a few minutes aside for yourself to rest and recharge.

Setting the scene

When giving your partner a comforting hand or foot massage, it is important to put a little effort into creating the right atmosphere. Although it is possible to offer a massage in just about any situation, attention to small details can transform a simple massage into a truly pampering and memorable experience. You will reap the benefits too – massaging in a warm and tranquil setting can be calming, revitalizing and incredibly rewarding.

Set aside time

Do not give a massage if you feel tired, rushed or bad tempered – as you will both end up feeling even more fraught. Make sure that you can spare the time to concentrate fully on giving the massage and the recipient's needs. And, if necessary, reassure your massage partner that you do not need to be elsewhere and are only too pleased to give a massage. It may be a good idea to

have a clock to hand and set a time limit of, say, 20 minutes, so you both know what to expect and are not concerned about being late for your next appointment. Choose the most favourable time of day, such as early evening when your massage partner will be able to relax afterward.

Create privacy

Depending on circumstances, close the door, switch on the answerphone, hang up a "do not disturb" sign and do all you can to make your massage partner feel safe and secure. Check that pets and children are settled and turn off – or shut out – as much television or traffic noise as possible. When you are confident that you will not be disturbed you will both find it easier to relax and enjoy the massage.

Prepare the room

Try to create a relaxing ambience. Lighting is important. Harsh, overhead or over-bright lighting can spoil the effect. If possible, use shaded, natural light or reduce the light level with side lamps or a dimmer switch. During the evening, you can enjoy the gentle glow of candlelight. An aromatic candle adds a sweet scent to the room. Check the room temperature too. Bare feet in a cold room can feel most uncomfortable. Have a blanket near-by in case your massage partner's body temperature drops as he or she relaxes. Ideally, the room should be warm, without being stifling, and well ventilated to allow the circulation of fresh air. Lay everything out so that you have all you need before the massage begins.

Dress for massage

Wear clothes that enable you to move freely and comfortably. Preferably something loose-fitting, short-sleeved and washable. Some oils can stain, so if you are concerned about your clothes wear an apron and wash it immediately afterward. Have your hair tied back from your face so it does not interfere with the massage; and remove your own and your massage partner's wrist-watch, bracelets, large rings or dangling earrings. Not only will they get in the way and possibly scratch your massage partner's skin, but the oil may damage them.

Choose music with care

At the start of the massage, offer your massage partner the choice of background music or silence. Some people prefer to have complete peace to gather their thoughts or drift off to some remote desert island. Or they may find it easier to relax to the sound of slow, soothing music. Most good music shops have a selection of tapes and CDs, specially composed for massage and relaxation. Choose something that you both enjoy – and play it quietly.

Get fresh

You will be in close proximity to your massage partner, especially when giving a hand massage, so personal hygiene is essential. Avoid wearing strong perfumes as this can be most off-putting and may negate the beneficial effects of essential oils. Wear clean clothes as the stale smell of food or drink can be most distasteful. Check your breath too – the odour of certain foods, cigarette smoke and coffee can linger for a long time. Clean your teeth or use a breath-freshening spray or gum. Wash your hands before massage, and be aware of keeping them smelling pleasant – wear rubber gloves when chopping onions or garlic, for example.

Warm and condition your hands

The warmth of your hands can help relax and reassure your massage partner, while the touch of cold hands can be quite a shock. Before you begin, rub your hands together briskly to generate warmth. Or, if you know they tend to get very cold, immerse them in warm water for a few minutes. Some people find having a hot drink prior to giving a massage helps raise their body tempera-ture and so warms their hands. Use hand cream regular-ly to soften your palms and smooth any rough patches. Try to keep your nails clean, trimmed and filed to avoid scratching the skin. It is best not to wear nail polish when massaging as this could chip off causing discomfort, and may trigger an allergic response in some people.

Discuss talking

At the start of the massage, explain to the recipient that massage is a way of offering some "me" time, to spend as he or she chooses, and not feel under any pressure to socialize. Your massage partner may simply want to relax and escape from life's stresses for a while. Or he or she may want to talk. Try to create an atmosphere where they feel psychologically comfortable enough to choose.

Check your posture

Comfort – both your massage partner's and your own – is essential for an effective massage. There are several possible positions for performing a hand or foot massage (see pages 64 and 81) so choose the one that is most comfortable for you. Check your massage partner feels well supported and relaxed. Experiment with different chairs, tables and cushions to find what suits you best. Good posture is important so you do not get too tired and suffer aches and pains. Twisting the spine can even lead to injury, so make sure the position you adopt will not force you to bend or stretch. Keep your body in direct alignment to the hand or foot being massaged, with your back straight but relaxed. Continue to be aware of your posture as you massage, and change positions and alternate hands, as necessary, to ensure your own comfort.

Plan your massage

Before attempting the routines on the following pages it is wise to read through the book first so you have an understanding of different massage techniques and are aware of hand and foot conditions. It is important to read

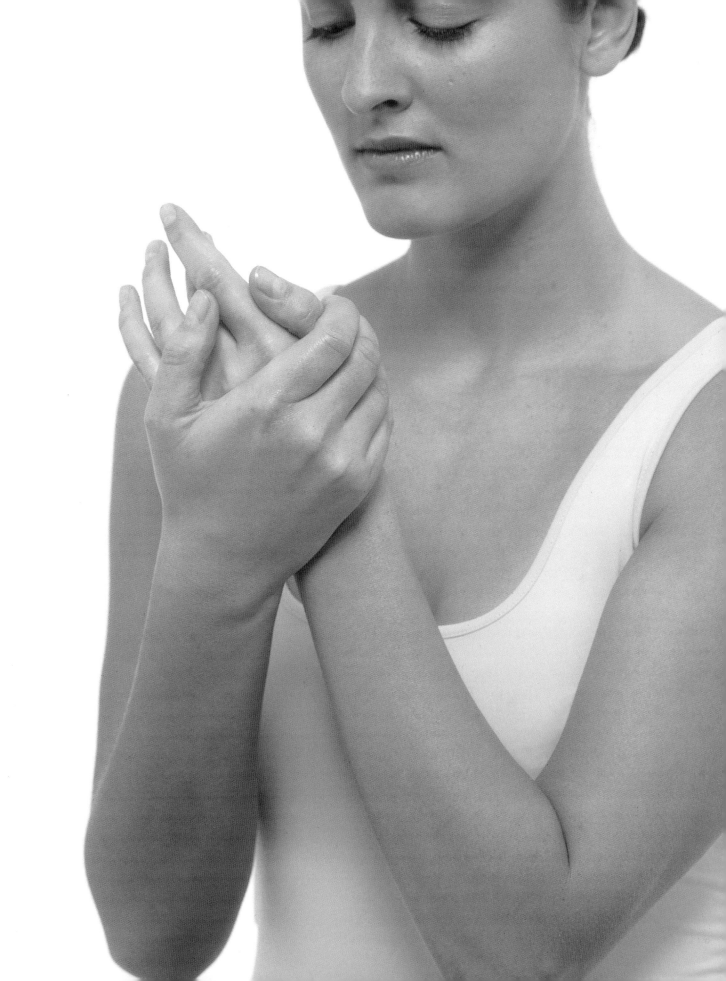

the sequences thoroughly – and practise some strokes on yourself to get a feel for them. Your massage partner may become rather irritated if you keep stopping and starting as you try to work out where your fingers and thumbs are supposed to be!

Be "centred"

During a massage you should "be there" for your massage partner. Put all your own concerns or worries out of your thoughts and be present in the moment. It is important to be able to detach yourself from your massage partner's emotions. This is often called being "centred" or "grounded" and is particularly important when massaging someone with deep-seated problems or a serious illness. Take a few moments to become calm and relaxed – physically and mentally. The following sequence may help:

1 Stand with your feet shoulder-width apart, feet firmly on the floor. Let your knees feel soft and your arms rest by your sides. Hunch your shoulders and then let them drop and relax – feel the tension easing. Grip your fingers tightly and then let go. Stand quietly for a minute or two, listening to the natural ebb and flow of your breathing.

2 Imagine your feet are like the golden roots of a tree growing deep into the ground, giving you strength and stability. Your body is firm and solid like the trunk of the tree. Your neck is light and relaxed and the top of your head is gently suspended from a delicate cord reaching upward into infinity. You are serene and confident with a sense of inner peace and calm.

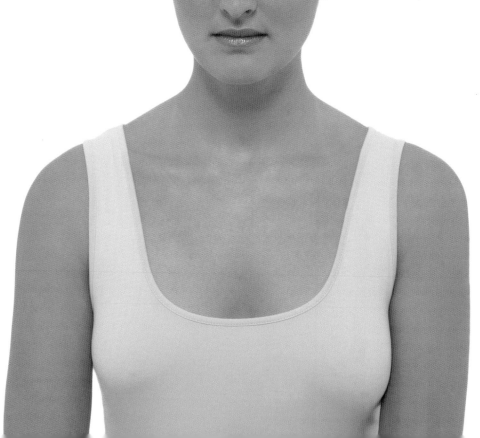

Breathing with your massage partner

When massaging, try to synchronize your breathing with that of your massage partner. This will help you focus your attention on your massage partner – both physically and mentally – and maximize the therapeutic potential of the massage. Sensitive people may pick up on a sense of detachment, for example, if you are mentally making a shopping list as you massage, and this can even seem disrespectful. At the very least, think about the foot or hand that you are massaging and tell it how much you love and respect it for all the hard work that it does. It can become like a mantra for you and soothe you mentally, too, as you massage.

Check hands and feet

At the start of your massage, always observe hands and feet – through vision and touch. Firstly, check for any conditions that may make massage inadvisable or where you need to take extra care (see pages 46–7). Then look for signs that may reflect your massage partner's state of health. These are not always accurate, but they do help to make you aware of the possibilities so you can adapt your massage accordingly or seek advice from your massage partner's doctor.

Colour

Check the colour of palms and soles, fingers and toes. A fleshy, pinkish colour indicates good circulation and balanced body systems. A very pale colour usually shows lack of blood flow to the extremities, which may be due to a drop in body temperature or general tiredness. Blue or purple hands and feet are a sign of poor circulation and, possibly, high levels of medication. While a red colour may indicate chronic stress and high blood pressure.

Temperature

Hands and feet should be pleasantly warm to touch. Coolness may indicate poor circulation and listlessness. When palms and soles feel very hot, this may be a sign of weight problems, high blood pressure, anxiety or burning anger.

Skin condition

Skin tissue should be soft and supple. Look for any signs of hard or cracked skin. This may indicate lack of adequate protection from detergents or the elements, poor posture or ill-fitting shoes.

Moisture

The skin on soles and palms should not feel too dry or too moist. If the skin is very dry this suggests a lack of fluid and poor circulation. If it is very damp it could indicate high levels of stress and anxiety, a weight problem or unsuitable footwear.

Flexibility of joints

If wrists and ankles are stiff, this may be associated with an injury or a joint condition such as arthritis. Special care should be taken when massaging.

Condition of nails

Healthy nails are pinkish in colour with a smooth surface and slight sheen. Poor circulation is usually indicated by a blue or purple tinge and brittle nails. Very thick, pitted nails may be a sign of a skin disorder, while horizontal ridges often appear a month or so after an illness or trauma.

Tension

Relaxed hands and feet indicate a relaxed person. If they feel tense, then chances are that your partner is too.

Our hands work for us continually, day in, day out. The many repetitive movements we perform can put strain, wear and tear on the tendons, ligaments and muscles.

5 *Hand* massage

Massage helps ease any build-up of tension, so increasing suppleness and preventing stiffness in the joints. Using a cream or oil helps moisturize and soften the skin, bringing an almost instant improvement in the appearance of even the most weather-beaten hands.

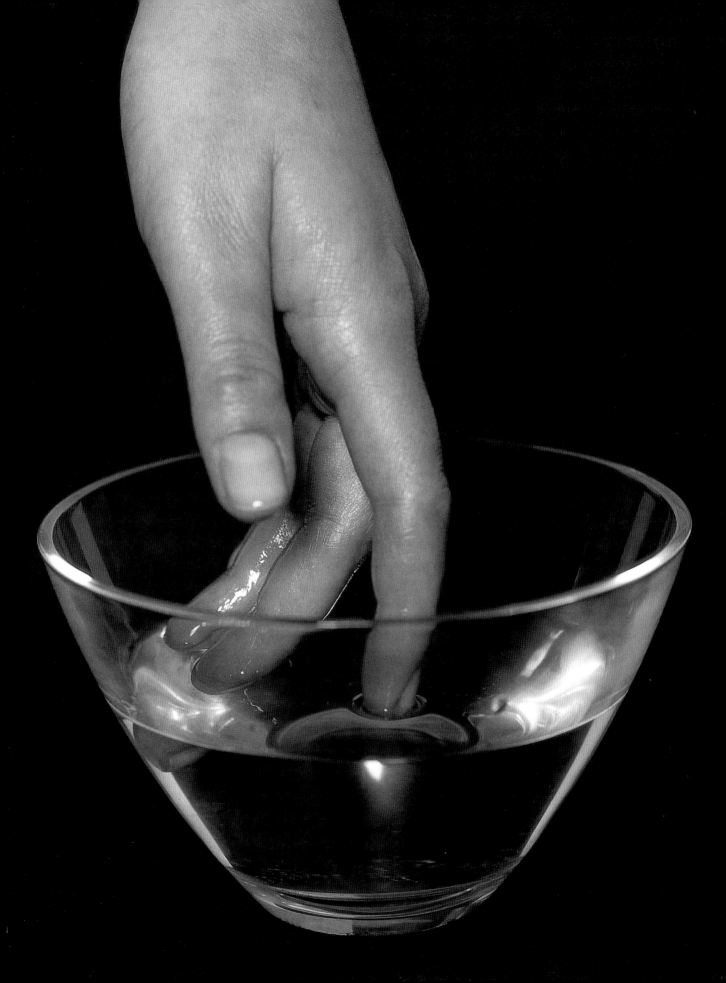

Self-massage
for tired and aching hands

This simple massage routine will help reduce muscle fatigue, relieve everyday aches and pains, encourage joint mobility and increase supplies of nourishing blood to improve the condition of the skin and nails. The use of oil or cream is optional, depending on when and where you massage your hands. If possible, sit on a chair and rest your elbows on a folded towel on a table or desk to offer extra support.

checklist

Preparation

- *Go to the loo*
- *Remove all jewellery on hands and wrists*
- *Roll sleeves up to the elbow*
- *Sit in a comfortable position*
- *Prepare a small amount of oil or cream (optional)*
- *Wash your hands*

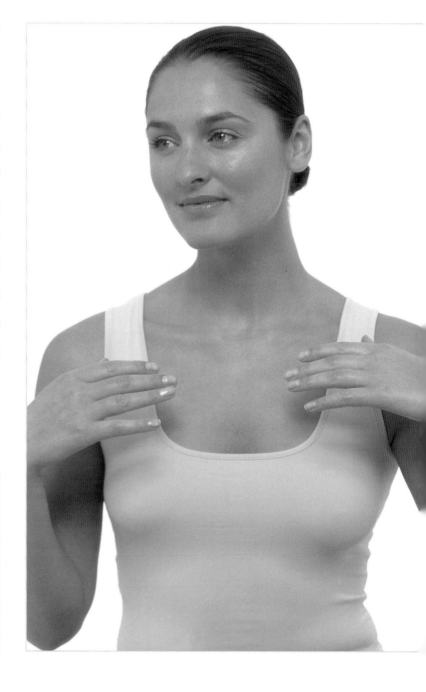

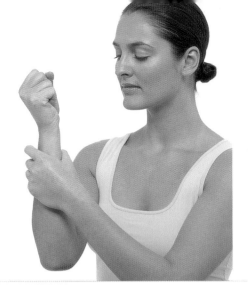

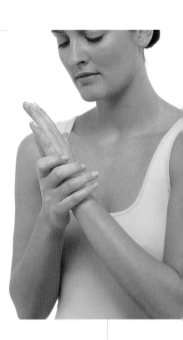

Practise these exercises whenever you need some speedy relief from nagging aches or want some natural warmth in cold weather.

WARM-UP EXERCISES

These simple exercises can help dissolve tension in tired hands and help boost circulation to cold fingers. Be cautious with these exercises if you have arthritis or another joint condition – seek the advice of your doctor or physiotherapist first.

1 Hold your hands at chest level and shake them from the wrist for a count of 10. Keep the movement loose and vigorous (left).

2 Now interlock your fingers. Stretch your arms out in front at shoulder height and then turn your hands so your palms face forward and thumbs down. Gently push the heels of your hands forward so that you feel a satisfying stretch from your wrist to your fingertips. Hold for the count of five. Release and repeat.

3 Support one wrist by firmly clasping it with the other hand. Now make your free hand into a soft fist and gently rotate the wrist in a clockwise direction (see above). Keep your supporting hand still – it does not play an active role. Do not force the movement, stay within a comfortable range of movement. Repeat three to five times. Now rotate your hand in the opposite direction, three to five times.

HAND RUBBING

This sequence helps improve the flow of blood to the hands and fingers so bringing nourishment and generating warmth in the area.

1 If you are using oil or cream, place an amount the size of a 5p piece in one of your hands. Now, rub your hands together so your palms and fingers are warm and well covered in lubricant. Massage your hands against each other – palm to palm, top of hand to palm and fingers to fingers. Really get them moving!

2 Place your palms together. Move them against each other in a circular motion with the heel of one hand exerting the pressure. Continue for about 20 seconds or longer. Repeat, with the other hand leading the action. Keep the movement slow and rhythmical.

These movements are useful for helping to spread oil or cream over your hands but they are also beneficial if you choose to do the massage dry – just pretend you are washing your hands with soap!

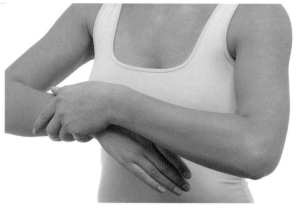
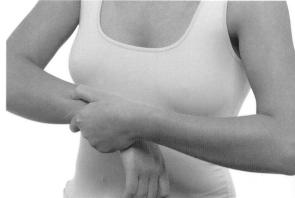

ARM STROKING

This sequence uses long, firm stroking movements to soothe the sensory nerve endings in your skin and warm your arms and hands.

1 With one forearm resting across your chest, or your elbow supported on a table or desk, use the palm and fingers of your other hand to stroke from the tips of your fingers to the elbow in a firm, smoothing action. When you reach the elbow, release the pressure and glide your hand back to the starting position. Continue until your forearm feels warm and relaxed, usually around 10 to 15 strokes.

2 Turn your forearm over and repeat the stroking action on the inner side of your arm.

• Keep your hand soft and relaxed so that it moulds naturally to the contours of your arm.

ARM KNEADING

These deeper, kneading strokes feel heavenly when you massage your own arms because you know exactly where to increase or decrease the pressure and speed of movement for best effect. Avoid massaging around the wrist if you have fragile bones or painful, swollen or arthritic wrists.

1 Rest one forearm across your chest, or support your elbow on a table or desk. Now grasp your forearm in the V between the thumb and forefinger of your free hand. The thumb is on top and fingers beneath. Make small circular movements with the flat of your thumb and the inside of your hand, moving from wrist to elbow. Maintain skin contact at all times. Increase the pressure on the upward half of the circle and decrease on the downward half. You will feel the skin moving against the underlying tissues and discover any areas of tension. When you reach the elbow, do a few small circles around it, then glide back down to the wrist to start again.

2 Repeat about six times to ensure the whole outer forearm is covered. Calm the area with some soothing strokes as shown in "Arm stroking".

3 Turn your arm over and repeat these circular movements on the inside of your forearm. Repeat six times and finish with "Arm stroking".

• Relax and feel the tensions of the day being released as you ease out the tension in these trouble spots. Push the tired feeling away.

tip

Keep focussing on your breathing as you massage your arms and hands. Try to let go of everyday stress for a few minutes – take some deep, calming breaths to help relieve any mental and physical tensions.

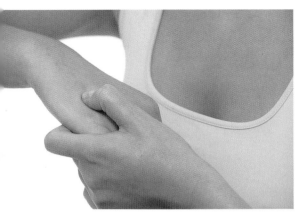

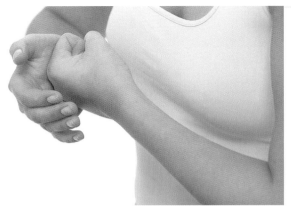

HAND KNEADING

This sequence feels wonderful when your hands tend to ache through over-use or general tiredness. Use a comfortably firm pressure.

1 Support your hand, palm downward, in the fingers of your other hand. Now place your thumb between the knuckles at the base of your little finger and ring finger. Use the fleshy pad of your thumb to stroke deeply and evenly in a straight line down the groove between the tendons, working toward the wrist. When your thumb reaches the wrist, release the pressure and glide back to the starting point. Repeat. Do the same movement along the other grooves on the top of your hand, finishing with the groove between the thumb and index finger.

2 With hands held in the same position, use the pad of your thumb to make small circular kneading movements down the groove between the little finger and ring finger. Maintain skin contact at all times, feeling for any areas of tension. As you massage, be aware of increasing the pressure on the upward half of the circle and decreasing it on the downward half. Repeat twice. Repeat along the other grooves on the top of your hand, finishing with the groove between the thumb and index finger.

3 Complete the sequence with some gentle stroking over the top of your hand.

• You may need to adjust your hand position to massage effectively.

PALM KNEADING

This is an instinctive massaging movement that you may already use when your hands feel weary. Enjoy the wonderful sense of relief as you target taut and over-worked muscles – but be cautious when massaging the wrist as the bones are very delicate. Avoid working on the wrist if you have fragile bones or painful, swollen or arthritic wrists.

1 Turn your hand over to work the palm. With your fingers supporting the back of your hand, use the fleshy pad of your thumb to make deep, circular movements over the whole of the palm and inner wrist. Pay special attention to the muscular pad at the base of the thumb. Start gently and slowly increase the pressure to get it right for you. Continue until you have covered your whole palm.

2 Now make your massaging hand into a fist and use your knuckles to knead the palm of the other hand. Alternatively, use the heel of your hand.

• We all hold tension in different places in our arms and hands. So, once you have learnt the basic movements, vary the routine and moves to suit your own personal needs. Experiment to find the most effective movements. You will know when you hit the spot!

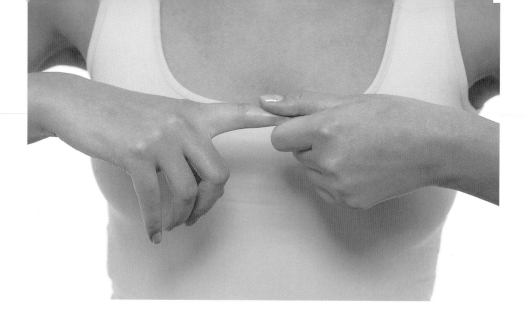

FINGER STRETCH

This sequence of movements will help increase blood circulation in your fingers and improve flexibility. Avoid if you have painful, swollen or arthritic fingers.

1 Hold the little finger of your right hand between the thumb and forefinger of your left hand. Curl your left hand around the little finger. Now gently squeeze and massage along the finger with a circular pressure. Move from the base of the finger to the tip.

2 When your hand reaches the tip of the finger, glide back down to the starting point. Now gently pull to give the whole finger a glorious stretch.

3 Release your grip and slide your hand to the top of the finger in one long, continuous movement. Allow your fingers to float away from the tip.

4 Repeat this sequence, working on each of your other fingers and thumb in turn.

- *Try this exercise to warm cold hands in the winter.*

FINGER TAPPING

These soft tapping movements help to stimulate sensory nerve endings in the skin, which have an energizing effect throughout the whole body.

1 Rest your right hand on a table or your knees, palm facing downward. Now use the flat of your fingers on your left hand to tap the back of the hand and fingers with light, rapid movements. Keep your wrists flexible and allow your fingers to bounce back as soon as they land on the skin.

2 Turn your hand over and continue springy movements across the palm and fingers.

3 Complete the sequence with some gentle stroking to calm the sensory nerve endings.

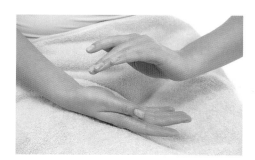

FINAL FLOURISH

Complete your hand massage by repeating "Arm stroking". On the return stroke, make the movement progressively lighter and slower, with your fingertips floating from the end of your fingers. Enjoy the soothing sense of release.

Soothing
hand massage

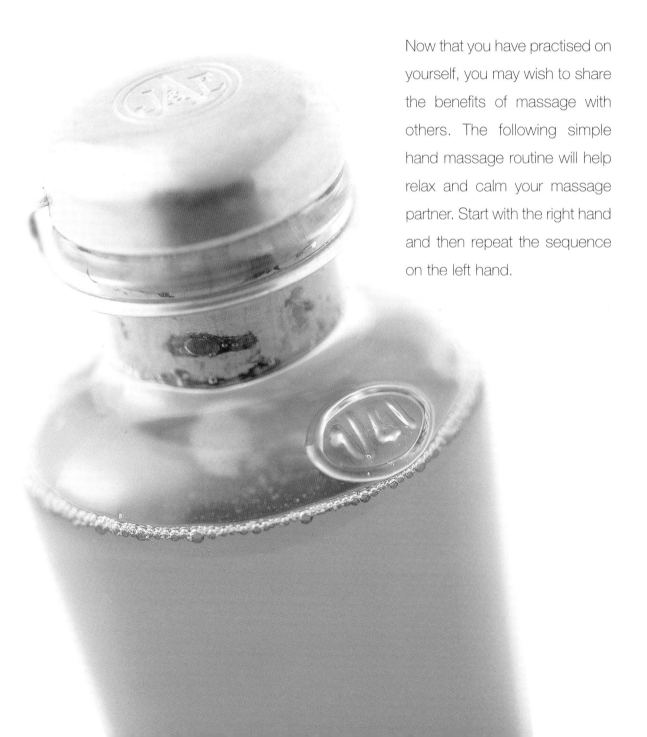

Now that you have practised on yourself, you may wish to share the benefits of massage with others. The following simple hand massage routine will help relax and calm your massage partner. Start with the right hand and then repeat the sequence on the left hand.

checklist
Things you will need

- Small pillow or cushion.
- Small table (optional).
- Two chairs.
- Suitable oil or cream in a small container (see Chapter Three).
- Wooden or plastic spatula for cream
- Two small towels.
- Paper towels to wipe your hands and absorb any spillage.
- Soft background music (optional).
- Blanket (optional).
- Clock (optional).
- Cologne (optional).
- Cotton wool (optional).

checklist
Advise your massage partner to:

- Go to the loo.
- Remove any rings, wristwatches or bracelets.
- Roll sleeves up to the elbow.
- Wash hands. Alternatively, clean them with wipes or cotton wool with a few drops of cologne.
- Tell you about any medical conditions that may affect your massage (see page 46). Ask about allergies and offer a choice of oil or cream.
- Try different positions to ensure you are both comfortable.
- Join you in breathing slowly and deeply, concentrating your thoughts on the massage that you are about to receive and give.

checklist
Things to do

- Dress in comfortable, washable clothes.
- Reduce the lighting.
- Check the room is warm and free from draughts.
- Arrange some privacy. Ensure that you will not be disturbed for the next 20 minutes or so. Switch on the answerphone or unplug the telephone.
- Wash your hands. Check that your nails are short, smooth and clean. Remove any jewellery that may interfere with the massage.
- Warm your hands by rubbing them briskly together. Do a few mobility exercises (see page 116–9) to help release any tension. Massage can make your own hands ache!

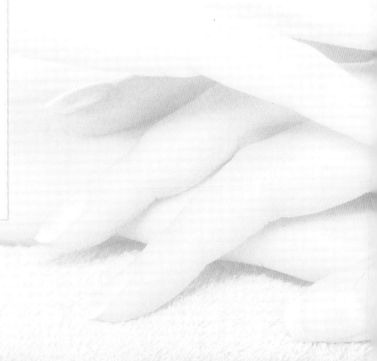

Getting prepared

Before you begin a massage, make sure those you massage know what to expect and are aware of the benefits. Give them the chance to ask any questions that may arise.

Talk it through

You may also like to ask whether they have had a hand massage before. If so, discuss any movements that they particularly liked or disliked. They may have some suggestions of their own. Use this time to discreetly assess, through looking and feeling, the condition of your massage partner's hand. Think about temperature, skin texture and colour (see page 55). Feel for any tension in the hand and check the condition of the nails. Check for any cuts, swollen joints or varicose veins (see page 46).

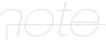

Hand massage brings you into close personal contact with your massage partner. You will be entering each other's personal space and this may feel a little uncomfortable at first. Be sensitive to your partner's reaction.

Get comfortable

Comfort is vital to relaxation. It is well worth spending a little time getting into a suitable position so you can massage without stretching or straining. You should both be able to move freely so that you can maintain a good posture during the massage. Depending on circumstances you may choose from the following:

Hand position one

You can sit facing each other. Cover a small cushion with a towel and place it on a small table between you, or on your lap. Rest your massage partner's hand on the cushion for the massage. Your feet, and those of your massage partner, should be placed firmly on the floor or small stool, ankles uncrossed. This is a good position for maintaining eye contact, but do be prepared to have your movements closely watched.

Hand position two

You can sit side by side. Your massage partner may choose to sit in a chair with one hand resting on a pillow on their lap or the armrest. Check the angle so you can work in comfort. Alternatively, if your massage partner is bedridden, you can easily massage the hands while they rest on a pillow on the side of the bed. This position is especially useful when massaging elderly or ill people. The disadvantage is that you will have to move your chair so you can massage each hand in comfort.

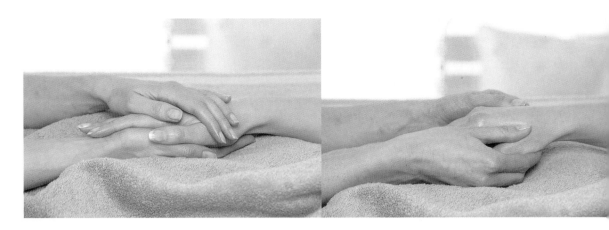

HOLDING THE HAND

*Simply holding your massage partner's hand in a caring way pro-
vides reassurance and comfort at the start of the massage. It
offers a moment of peace and stillness that helps establish a bond
and allows you both to let go of tension and relax into the experience. It is important not to rush this preliminary hold.*

1 Begin with your massage partner's hand facing
palm downward. Place one of your hands
beneath and the other on top, so that the hand is
cradled in the warmth and security of your palms.
Maintain optimum contact by using the whole surface area of palms and fingers.

2 Hold for a minute. At this stage you may like to
ask your massage partner to close her eyes and
take some deep breaths, in and out, to encourage relaxation. Remind your massage partner to
try to "let go" of her everyday hassles and simply
enjoy being pampered.

3 Release your hold very gradually by sliding
your hands toward the fingertips, and gently and
slowly drawing away.

tip

> *Look out for areas of dry skin. Massage the
> cream or oil into these patches to moisturize
> and soften the hands.*

GENTLE STRETCH

*This stretching movement is wonderfully soothing, especially
for tired, aching hands.*

1 Place some oil or cream in the palm of one of
your hands. As a rough guide, an amount the size
of a 5p coin is a good starting point. If you use too
much you may find your hands slipping and sliding over the skin. You can easily top it up during
the massage if your hands are large or your massage partner's skin is very dry. Rub your hands
together so that the palms and fingers are warm
and well covered in oil or cream.

2 With your partner's hand facing palm downward, place a hand on either side with fingers
curled underneath and your thumbs on top. Cup
the sides of your massage partner's hand in your
hands. Now draw your thumbs firmly out to the
sides to achieve a pleasant rolling and stretching
action over the back of her hand. Use the whole
length of your thumbs to gain maximum benefit.

3 When your thumbs reach the sides of the
hand, hold for a count of three, then release and
repeat twice more.

• *Work on the top of the hand, avoid pressing on your
partner's fingers.*

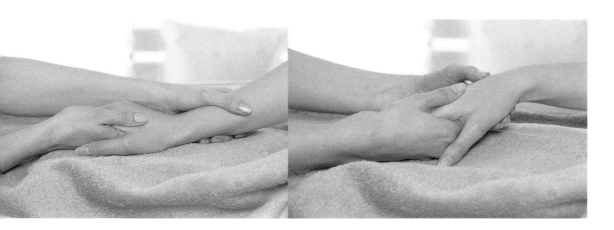

WARMING UP

This sequence uses confident, sweeping movements to relax your massage partner and stimulate blood circulation. Use these warm-up strokes as a way of becoming more familiar with the feel of your partner's skin beneath your hands.

1 With your massage partner's palm facing downward, place one hand beneath to offer support – in a loose "shaking hands" position. Now sweep your other hand firmly up from the finger tips along the upper side of the arm toward the elbow in a long, steady stroke. Work with your whole hand and keep it soft and relaxed so it moulds to the shape of her arm. Glide around the elbow and return with a lighter pressure to the fingers. Repeat around six to 10 times.

2 Turn your massage partner's arm slightly and change your working hand to perform these gliding strokes along the inside of the forearm. Sweep lightly into the elbow crease before returning to the wrist. Repeat six to ten times.

3 Complete the sequence by gently holding your partner's hand for a few seconds.

• *Ensure that any dry skin is well lubricated with oil or cream.*

STROKING THE BACK OF THE HAND

These rhythmical strokes help warm and soften the hand so that it is well prepared for the subsequent movements. The bones of the hand are very delicate, so maintain a light pressure.

1 With the palm of your massage partner's hand facing downward, wrap your hands around it, thumbs on top and fingers beneath. Use the pads of your thumbs to make alternate strokes along the top of the hand, working from the fingers to the wrist. Your thumbs move one after the other in a wave-like flowing motion.

2 When your thumbs reach the wrist, lessen the pressure and, without losing contact, slide them back to the starting position. Repeat the sequence six times to cover the whole of the top of the hand.

• *Spend longer on these movements if you sense that your massage partner needs soothing comfort.*

tip

Synchronize your breathing with that of your massage partner. Focus on your partner. Thinking about other things may well convey a feeling of detachment.

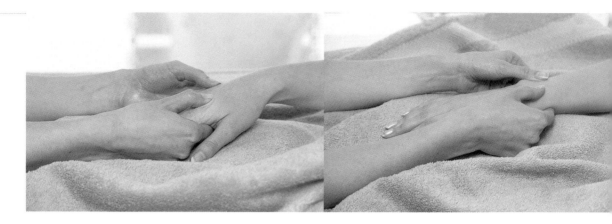

KNEADING THE BACK OF THE HAND

This sequence of movements is effective in releasing muscular tension and tiredness in hands. The pressure should be satisfying but not painful.

1 With the palm of your massage partner's hand facing downward, place your fingers beneath and thumbs on top as in the previous movement. Use the pads of your thumbs to make alternate strokes along the groove between the tendons of the little finger and third finger. Work from the knuckles to the wrist. Begin with a fairly firm but comfortable pressure and gradually release the pressure as your thumb reaches the wrist. Return with a light pressure, still maintaining contact. Repeat. Now repeat this stroking action along each of the grooves on the top of the hand, including between the thumb and forefinger.

2 Return your hands to the starting position and use the fleshy pads of your thumbs to make alternate small circular movements along the groove between the little finger and third finger. Move toward the wrist, maintaining contact with the skin. Repeat. Now repeat the movement working rhythmically along each of the grooves on the top of the hand.

3 Finish with some soothing stokes over the top of the hand working toward the wrist.

• You will need to change working hands to perform this effectively, but always maintain a good support and never lose contact.

WRIST RELEASE

Wrists are so neglected. Your massage partner will feel the tension leaving her wrists with your gentle touch. Avoid this movement if a massage partner has fragile bones or painful, swollen or arthritic wrists.

1 Start with your hands on either side of your massage partner's hand, as in the previous movement. Place your fingers beneath her inner wrist and your thumbs on top. Now make small, alternating circles with the pads of both thumbs over the back of the wrist. The movement should be fairly slow and rhythmical with a comfortably firm pressure. Make around 15 to 20 small circles.

2 Now change the movement to a gentle fanning action using both thumbs to stroke upward from the wrist in an arc shape. Your thumbs come gently off the skin at the sides of the arm about 5 cm (2 in) about the wrist. Thumbs can work together or alternately in a rhythmic flowing action. Repeat around six times.

• Do not press too firmly as the bones in the wrist are very delicate.

tip

Keep your massage as fluid and rhythmical as possible, flowing smoothly between movements. Try not to stop and start.

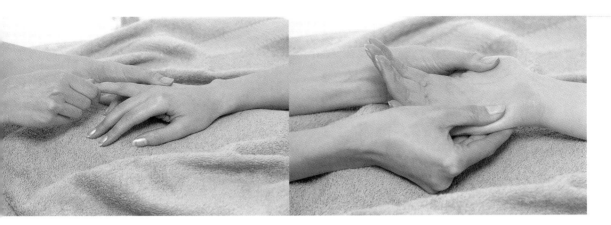

FINGER WORK

This sequence of movements helps maintain suppleness and range of movement in the fingers. It also helps relax and warm cold hands. Avoid if the person has painful, swollen or arthritic joints. Change working hands as necessary.

1 Clasp the hand, palm downward, with one hand. With your other hand, hold your massage partner's little finger between your thumb and forefinger. The finger should be well supported from the base. Rotate the whole finger three times in a clockwise direction, and then three times in an anti-clockwise direction. Ask your massage partner not to help with the rotation but to "let go" and allow you to do the movement instead.

2 Now place the little finger between your thumb and forefinger so that it is supported in the turn of your fingers. Maintaining this position, use the pad of your thumb to make gentle circular movements along the finger, working from base to tip.

3 When your thumb reaches the tip of your massage partner's finger, push your thumb and fingers downward in a firm stroking movement. Hold, so that the whole finger is enclosed in your hand. Now release the pressure slightly and draw your hand in the opposite direction, allowing it to slide off the tip of the finger in a gentle pulling, stretching action. Repeat the sequence.

4 Repeat the same sequence of movements on each finger in turn, finishing with the thumb.

PALM STRETCH

This sequence helps stretch and soften constricted muscle fibres in the palm, so making the palm more relaxed and pliant.

1 Sandwich your massage partner's hand between your two palms and turn it over so that the palm faces upward. Make the movement definite so that you are in control.

2 Now rest the back of your massage partner's hand on your fingers and place your thumbs on the palm, pointing toward the wrist. Push your thumbs gently outward to the sides to spread and stretch the palm. Use your thumbs to hold the stretch for a count of five, then release and repeat twice.

• *This is the reverse action to "Gentle Stretch" (page 66).*

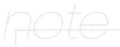

Be aware of your massage partner's body language. Around 70 per cent of all communication is by means of non-verbal massages and gestures. Take note of any flinching or stiffening, which may indicate discomfort or unease. Similarly look for signs of pleasure such as relaxed breathing. Adapt your massage accordingly.

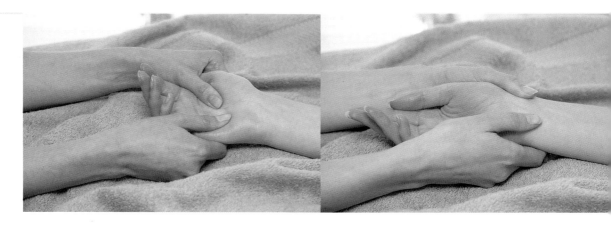

PALM STROKING AND KNEADING

These movements ease tension in taut muscles in the palm. Some people call this "walking in the palm".

1 With your massage partner's palm facing upward, wrap your hands around the sides of the hand, fingers underneath and thumbs in the palm. Use the pads of your thumbs to make small alternate stroking movements covering the whole palm. Work from fingers toward wrist. Thumbs work one after the other in a wave-like flowing action. Glide over the surface of the skin with a smoothing, nurturing touch.

2 Now start kneading the palm. Make alternate, circular movements with the fleshy pads of your thumbs, increasing the pressure on the upward half of the circle and decrease on the downward half. Keep the movement slow, firm and rhythmical with one thumb working after the other. Cover the whole of the palm, paying special attention to the muscular pad at the base of the thumb.

3 Follow this with some firm sliding strokes. Use the pads of your thumbs to make a fanning movement from the base of the fingers toward the wrist. Your thumbs move at the same time. As they slide off the hand at the sides of the wrist they return to the starting position and begin again. Repeat approx. 10 times.

4 Finish the sequence by repeating Step 1.

• The fleshy pad of the palm usually responds well to deep massage but check your pressure is comfortable as some areas may be tender.

INNER WRIST STROKING

This movement is surprisingly soothing and can have an almost hypnotic effect. Avoid this movement if the person has fragile bones or painful, swollen or arthritic wrists.

1 With your massage partner's hand remaining in the palm-upward position, rest your fingers on the back of the wrist and your thumbs on the inner wrist. Use the pads of your thumbs to make alternate, small circular movements with a light pressure. Cover the whole of the inner wrist.

2 Change the movement to a gentle fanning action using both thumbs to stroke upward from the wrist in an arc shape. Your thumbs come gently off the skin at the sides of the arm about 5 cm (2 in) about the wrist. Repeat six times.

• Maintain a good support and keep your pressure very light to avoid causing pain or discomfort around the delicate bones of the wrist.

note

During a hand massage make every effort to ensure your partner feels nurtured, cossetted and secure. Try not to rush any movements. Gentle, unhurried, rhythmical strokes are soothing and relaxing for you both.

WRIST ROTATIONS

These gentle circling movements help to mobilize wrist joints and prevent the common problems of stiffness and swelling. Make the movement firm and controlled but do not force the action. Be cautious if your massage partner has arthritis, or has had a previous wrist injury.

1 For this movement your massage partner's forearm is slightly raised. Use one hand to gently support the lower arm – avoid gripping tightly. Interlock the fingers of your free hand with those of your massage partner to ensure a firm, supportive hold. Alternately, clasp your hands as though shaking each other's hands.

2 Now slowly rotate the wrist. Repeat three times in a clockwise direction and three times in an anticlockwise direction.

3 Gently lay down the arm and hand and slowly release your fingers.

tip

Feel the range of movement in your partner's wrist and remain within her own personal limits. You may find that your partner tries to help with the movement. If so, ask her to look away or close her eyes so that you can control the action.

FINISHING TOUCH

Complete the massage with some soothing strokes to relax mind, body and spirit.

1 With your massage partner's palm facing downward, place one hand beneath it to offer warmth and reassurance. Repeat the same soothing strokes used at the beginning of the massage in the "warming up" sequence to massage the hand and arm. Allow the strokes to become progressively lighter and slower.

2 Now use the tips of the fingers on your free hand to stroke the top of your massage partner's hand with a feather-like touch as though stroking a cat. Work from wrist to fingertips, allowing your fingers to float from the end of your massage partner's fingertips.

3 Place your free hand on top of your massage partner's hand to enclose it securely in the warmth of your palms for around 10 seconds, or longer if you wish. Release your hold and slowly draw your hands away.

• *Cover your massage partner's hand with a towel and repeat the routine on the other hand.*

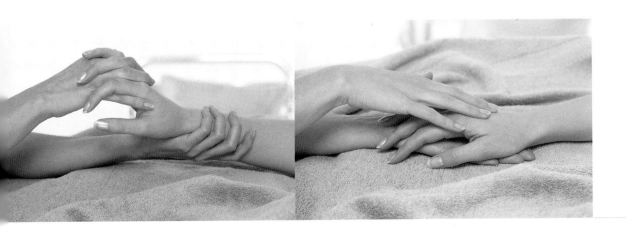

Feet contain thousands of tiny sensory nerve endings, making them among the most sensitive areas of the whole body. Your massage can be adapted to stimulate or soothe these nerve endings and thus energize or relax yourself and your massage partner.

6 Foot massage

A brisk massage can help to boost energy levels and restore a sense of well-being. A slower massage can be extremely relaxing and offer comfort and reassurance during a stressful or difficult time.

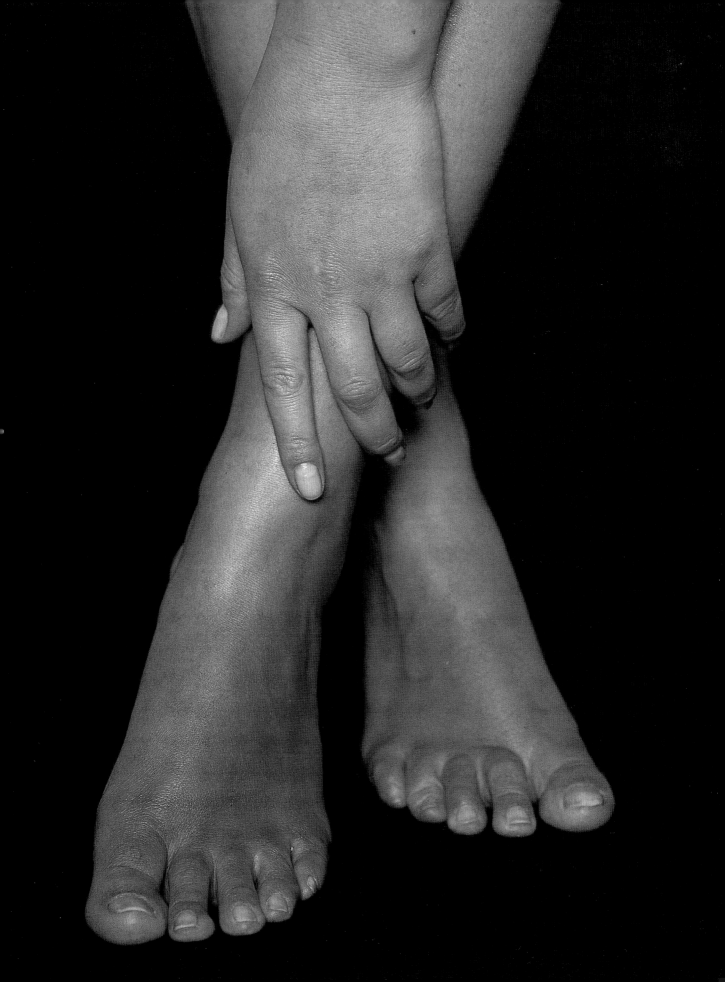

Self foot-massage
for boosting circulation

If you suffer the miseries of cold feet, then try this quick and effective self-help routine. It can be done wherever you are – at home or at work. You may choose to use a nourishing oil or cream, but many of the strokes are just as effective performed dry without even removing your socks or tights. You need to be able to reach your foot comfortably, either sitting on the floor, a chair or a bed. Experiment to find the most suitable position for you.

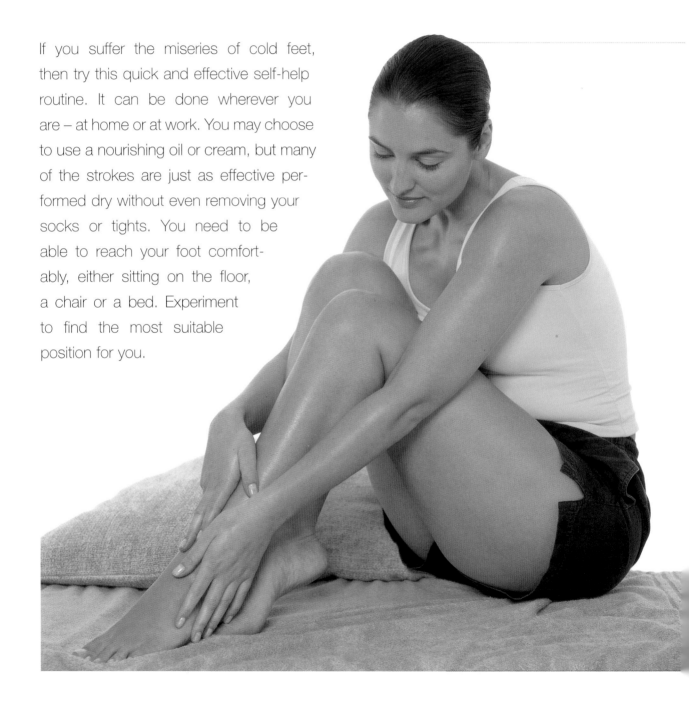

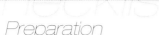

Preparation

- *Remove all jewellery on hands, feet, wrists and ankles.*
- *Remove shoes.*
- *Sit in a comfortable position.*
- *Prepare a small amount of oil or cream (optional, see Chapter Three).*
- *Go to the loo.*
- *Wash your hands in warm water – they need to be warm before you begin.*

WARMING START

Give your circulation a kick-start with these smooth, sweeping strokes. A firm, confident pressure will improve poor blood and lymph circulation in the feet and lower legs.

1 If you are using oil or cream, roll up your trouser legs and remove socks or tights. (This is best done at the start when your hands are dry.) Place some oil or cream, around the size of a 10p is usually sufficient, in the palm of one of your hands. Rub your hands together so they are warm and well covered in lubricant.

2 With your knee bent, stroke both hands up your leg moving from the ankle toward the knee in a slow, rhythmical, flowing action. Keep your hands open and soft, maintaining as much contact with the palms and fingers as possible. Imagine your hands are plasticine or playdough and mould them to the contours of your legs.

3 Gradually increase the pressure using long, even and confident strokes on the upward movement toward the knee. Lessen the pressure at the knee and glide back down the sides of the leg to the starting position.

4 Work the back and front of the lower leg until it feels warm and relaxed.

- *Continue for as long as it feels good – and it does!*

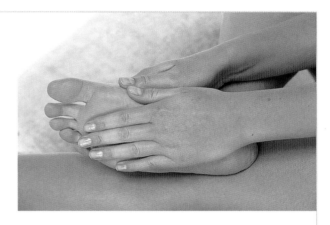

FOOT STROKING

Now that your leg is warm, turn your attention to the foot. Rest the ankle of one foot on a towel across the thigh of the other leg. Alternatively, if you are sitting on the floor you may prefer to rest on a cushion.

1 Sandwich your foot between the palms of your hands and, with both hands moving simultaneously, stroke from the toes to the heel in one long continuous movement. Repeat three times.

2 With hands held in the same position, start moving the flat of your hands in large circles, one on top and one beneath, rather like the wheels of a train.

3 Finish the sequence by holding your foot between the palms of your hands, fingers facing toward the toes. Draw your hands down your foot and slide very lightly right off the end of your toes. Repeat three times.

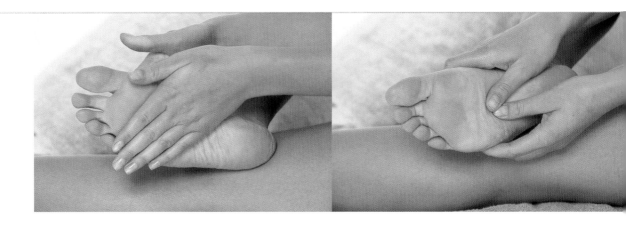

FOOT RUB

Rubbing your feet is a natural response when we feel chilly as it helps to generate warmth. – and feels wonderful. The pressure should be fairly firm to stimulate the local blood circulation and warm and invigorate your whole body.

1 With your foot sandwiched between the palms of your hands, rub briskly over the surface of the skin using short, stimulating movements back and forth in any direction. You will find that one hand naturally moves forward as the other moves backward. Your wrists stay flexible, fingers held quite straight. Cover your whole foot, including your toes, heel and ankle.

2 Finish with some soothing strokes over the whole foot.

• *Keep your hands moving so you do not stay in the same spot for too long.*

SOLE FANNING

This movement feels best when the pressure is comfortably firm. Relax and enjoy the sensation.

1 Support your foot in both hands, fingers on top of the foot and thumbs meeting on the arch of the foot. Now press with the pads of your thumbs and, with one long, sweeping fan-like movement, push them upward to the base of your toes and out to the sides of the foot. Your thumbs should stay fairly stiff and in contact with the skin as you sweep them up to form a curved T-shape.

2 Maintain an even pressure on the upward movement and then skim over the skin to return to the starting position. Repeat four times.

note

The sole of the foot is very sensitive to touch. Notice how gentle strokes soothe the whole body whilst brisker strokes have a more stimulating effect.

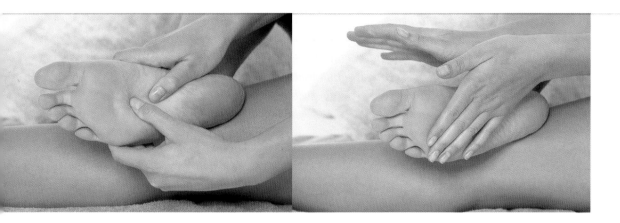

SOLE SEARCHING

Use these kneading movements to target the tension hot-spots in the sole of your foot. You will know exactly where to work for the best results. These techniques help to loosen muscles, ease aches and pains, and improve poor circulation.

1 With hands held in the same position as above, use the pads of your thumbs to make small circular movements over the whole of the sole of your foot and around your heel. Your thumbs work simultaneously, exerting a deep but comfortable pressure – feel the sense of relief as you knead this area.

2 Now support the top of the foot with one hand and make a loose fist with your free hand. Firmly rotate your fist over the sole of the foot using your knuckles to make small circular tension-releasing movements.

3 Complete the sequence by soothing any slight discomfort caused by deep kneading with some gentle stroking around the foot.

FOOT TAPPING

This is an energizing, uplifting movement that stimulates the blood circulation to your feet and makes you feel good all over. Avoid this action over inflamed areas or corns.

1 Lightly tap your toes with the flat of your hands, one hand moving after the other in the same rapid, rhythmical way as playing a percussion instrument. Keep your wrists loose and allow your fingers to bounce back as soon as they land on the skin. Begin slowly and then gradually increase your speed so the movement is energetic and springy.

2 Repeat this light striking action over the top and sole of the foot.

3 Follow this invigorating movement with some gentle stroking to soothe the area.

• *Try using the back or side of your hand to tap the sole of the foot.*

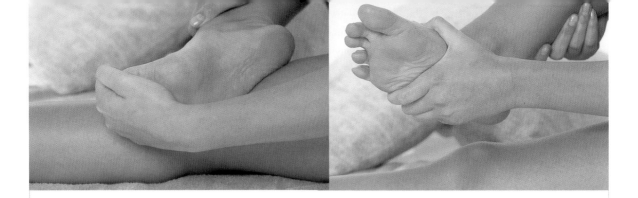

TOE STRETCHING AND CIRCLING

If your toes tend to feel the cold, then practise this sequence regularly to help loosen joints and maintain good circulation to the extremities. If you have painful, swollen or arthritic joints in your toes, consult your doctor or physiotherapist before doing this exercise.

1 Supporting your foot in one hand, hold all five toes in your other hand. Clasp the toes firmly with the palm of your hand on the ball of the foot, fingers curled over the toes and pointing along the top of the foot toward the ankle. Gently push against your toes to bend them toward your leg. Hold for a count of six. Release. Repeat four times, keeping the movement slow and controlled.

2 With hands held in the same position, grasp your toes firmly and gently rotate all five toes at once. Begin by moving them in a clockwise direction. Repeat six times. Now reverse the movement so they are circled in the other direction. Repeat six times.

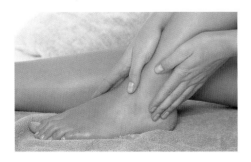

ANKLE CIRCLING

A foot massage is not complete without ankle rotations. This simple movement helps maintain flexibility and prevents stiffness and is also a most effective circulation-boosting exercise. If you have painful, swollen or arthritic ankles, consult your doctor or physiotherapist first.

1 Support your leg with one hand placed just above the ankle. Clasp the foot with the other hand. Maintaining a firm hold, use your hand to rotate your ankle in a clockwise direction. Keep the movement definite and controlled, aiming to achieve your full range of movement – but do not force the movement. Repeat five times.

2 Circle the ankle in the other direction five times.

• Make ankle circling part of your daily routine. You will find that your ankle mobility gradually starts to increase.

FINAL STROKES

By now your foot should feel warm and revitalized. To complete your massage, soothe the nerve endings with some slow stroking.

1 Stroke your hands firmly from your toes up to your ankles. Continue the stroke up to your knee, if you wish.

2 Cover your whole foot and lower leg with light, calming strokes using the tips of your fingers.

3 Now hold your foot between your two palms. Stay still and feel the warmth of your hands against your foot. Slowly release the hold and draw your hands away.

• Cover your foot with a towel to keep warm and repeat the sequence on the other foot.

Reviving
foot massage

A foot massage can also help to refresh tired feet, get rid of aches, keep joints flexible and boost blood circulation. Try this sequence on a massage partner, varying the depth and speed of strokes as appropriate to the mood and occasion. Begin with the right foot and then repeat the sequence of movements on the left foot.

checklist
Things you will need

- Small pillow or cushion.
- Two chairs, small table and/or cushions depending on position.
- Suitable oil or cream in a small container (see Chapter Three).
- Wooden or plastic spatula (for cream).
- Two small towels.
- Paper towels to wipe your hands and absorb spillage.
- Soft background music (optional).
- Blanket (optional).
- Clock (optional).
- Cologne (optional).
- Cotton wool (optional).
- Mirror (optional).
- Shoehorn (optional).

checklist
Advise your massage partner to:

- Wear loose, comfortable clothing. Trousers are rolled up for lower leg massage.
- Remove any foot rings or ankle chains.
- Tell you about any conditions that may affect your massage (see page 46). (Ask your massage partner about allergies and offer a choice of oils or creams.)
- Go to the loo.
- Try different positions to ensure maximum comfort for you both.
- Join you in breathing deeply and slowly, allowing your thoughts to centre on the massage time you are about to share.

checklist
Things to do

- Dress in comfortable, washable clothes.
- Reduce the lighting.
- Check the room is warm and free from draughts.
- Arrange to have privacy. Make sure that you will not be disturbed for the next half hour or so. Switch on the answerphone.
- Remove any jewellery that may interfere with the massage.
- Wash your hands.
- Check your nails are short, smooth and clean. Cover any cuts or abrasions with sticking plaster.
- Warm your hands by rubbing them briskly together. Do a few mobility exercises (see page 116–9) to help release any tension.

Getting prepared

Some people feel a little strange about having their feet massaged. They may be concerned that their feet are ugly or smelly, or that your touch will tickle. So, before starting your massage, explain exactly what is going to happen and outline briefly some of the benefits.

Talk it through

Give your massage partner the chance to ask any questions and reassure him or her that you will stop if any movements are painful or uncomfortable.

Be comfortable

There is a temptation to launch straight into a massage without thinking about your position. It is often only half way through that you realize your back is aching and your partner is still unable to relax. So spend a little time and effort making sure that you are both comfortable, well supported and at the right angle for massage. Ideally, your back should be straight with your massage partner's feet at chest height to avoid muscle tension in your arms. You should be able to move freely and breathe easily. With some creative experimentation, you will find the ideal solution. Depending on circumstances, you may choose from the following:

Foot position one

Your massage partner lies on a bed or reclining chair with her feet at the foot. You sit on a lower chair or stool so that you face your massage partner and have easy access to the soles of the feet. Place a small cushion or rolled up towel beneath her knees so that the feet are in the most relaxed position. Make sure your massage partner feels comfortable and that her neck and back are well supported. Use extra pillows to prop her up if she chooses to sit in a semi-reclining position.

Foot position two

Your massage partner sits on a chair with her legs resting on a stool or small table of a similar height. Alternatively, she rests her feet on your lap. Place her feet on a cushion covered in a towel, knees slightly bent. You sit facing your massage partner on a chair, stool or cushion but do check your height and position so that you maintain a good posture and do not need to lean further forward than is comfortable. One drawback of this position is privacy – your massage partner may prefer to wear trousers or rest a towel over her lap.

Foot position three

Your partner rests against a pile of cushions on the floor. You kneel or sit cross-legged on the floor with your back against a wall or heavy piece of furniture. Your massage partner's feet rest on a cushion on your lap.

Cleaning up

It is perfectly natural to feel embarrassed at the possibility of having dirty or smelly feet – even if you have just walked straight out of the shower. So put your massage partner at ease by cleansing her feet. Use antiseptic or baby wipes or cotton wool with some cologne. Warn her that the wipes or cotton wool may feel a little chilly at first. Use separate pieces for each foot to avoid cross infection. While cleaning her feet, handle them with tenderness and care as though saying a gentle "hello" to them. Use the opportunity to assess their condition. Check temperature, skin texture, colour and tension. Look for any cuts, swollen joints, varicose veins or fungal infections (see Chapter Nine).

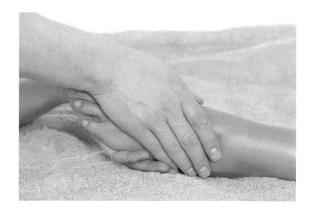

GREETING THE FEET

First impressions matter – and your first contact with your massage partner's feet sets the tone for the whole massage. Be confident and reassuring. Feel how the person's feet gradually soften and become more receptive to your touch.

1 Gently cradle your massage partner's right foot in both hands. Hold the foot securely with maximum skin-to-skin contact, so encouraging the foot to relax within the warmth and comfort of your palms.

2 Hold for a minute or two. You may like to ask your massage partner to take some deep breaths to help her relax and gain the optimum benefits from your massage. You can join in too. It is surprising how effective deep breathing can be in allowing you to let go of everyday tensions.

3 Release your hold by slowly drawing your hands away.

• *Do not be tempted to rush this initial hold. It helps inspire a feeling of trust from your partner.*

tip

Depending on your foot position, you may need to adapt some of the movements slightly to allow your arms and hands to move freely.

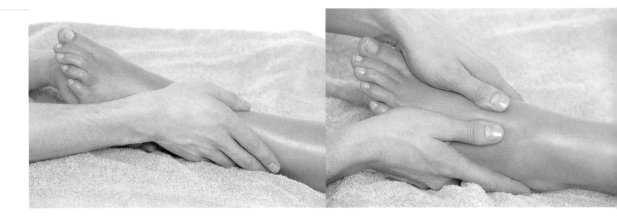

WARMING STROKES

This sequence of flowing strokes smoothes in the cream or oil, and warms and prepares the foot for massage.

1 Place some oil or cream in the palm of your hands. Around the size of a 10p coin is usually sufficient. Add more if the skin on your massage partner's feet are very dry but be careful not to over-do it or your hands will slip and slide. Rub your hands together so that your palms and fingers are warm and well covered in lubricant.

2 Now sandwich the right foot between your palms – one hand covering the top of the foot and the other on the sole. Place your hands in a prayer position so you obtain maximum skin-to-skin contact.

3 Slide your hands gently but firmly from the tips of the toes up toward the body. It may help to move your elbows out to the sides. When your hands reach the ankle, glide back with a lighter pressure down toward the toes, maintaining contact throughout. It is a smooth, rhythmical, sweeping action, following the contours of the foot. Your hands should be aiming to mould themselves to the foot.

4 If you choose, you can sweep the strokes right up to the knee, keeping a firmer pressure on the upward movement and gliding back down to the ankle.

5 Repeat several times until the foot feels warm and relaxed.

• *Cover your partner's other foot with a towel to keep it warm.*

OPENING THE FOOT

This is a wonderful stretching and releasing movement that helps ease the tension in tired and aching feet. Try it on yourself when you have been on your feet all day long.

1 Position your hands on either side of the foot – fingers on the sole and thumbs on the top of the foot. Now exert a slight pressure with your thumbs to stretch out the top of the foot and bring the sides toward you. As your thumbs move outward, feel the foot gently arching. Hold for a count of five and gently release.

2 Repeat three times, moving a little further down the foot each time.

• *Keep the pressure on the top of the foot, be careful not to press on your partner's toes.*

note

Your massage partner's feet deserve some care and respect. After all, it has been estimated that during an average lifespan most of us walk the equivalent of four times the circumference of the Earth! Every time we take a step we put around one and a quarter times our body weight on each foot. For most people this amounts to a total force of over one million pounds every day.

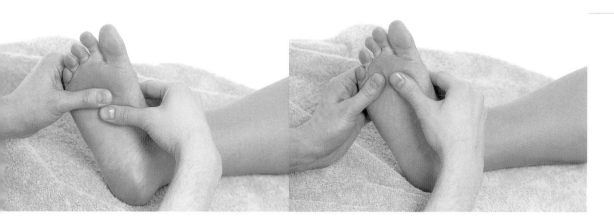

SOLE CRISS-CROSS

Firm massage movements on the sole of the foot can be really pleasurable. This deep stroking movement helps to ease tension and warm the sole of the foot. Try to maintain a slow, steady rhythm with even pressure.

1 Clasp the foot with both hands, your thumbs on the heel and fingers overlapping on top of the foot. Now, slide one thumb above the other in a criss-cross action toward either side of the foot. Your thumbs move with a firm pressure toward and past each other, moving simultaneously in opposite directions. Without losing contact with the skin, use this alternate back-and-forth action to move your hands up the foot so that the whole sole is covered.

2 Continue the criss-cross action moving down to the heel.

3 Repeat three times.

● *Try using different speeds. A slow action is very soothing while a brisker movement is invigorating.*

THUMB CIRCLES

This sequence works a little deeper, helping to stimulate blood circulation to the sole of the foot, so generating warmth and encouraging flexibility.

1 With your hands in the same position as the start of the previous movement, use the fleshy pads of your thumbs to make small circular movements over the sole of the foot. Your thumbs work simultaneously to rotate the skin against the underlying tissues. It is a rhythmical, kneading movement – press, lift, squeeze and release the flesh.

2 Work upward from the heel to the base of the toes in a smooth, continuous movement so that your thumbs do not leave the skin. Repeat these thumb circles so the entire sole is covered.

● *Keep checking the pressure with your partner as some areas of the foot may be a little tender.*

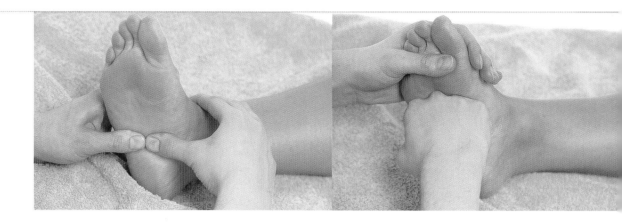

THUMB STROKING

This deep stroking sequence feels blissful after the previous kneading movement. You must be in a position where you can lean slightly backward and keep your back straight.

1 Hold the foot with both hands, fingers overlapping on top and thumbs on the ball of the foot. Mould your fingers to the foot so that it rests securely in your hand. Now make short, sweeping, downward movements with your thumbs. One thumb strokes after the other, in a rhythmical, wave-like movement.

2 Follow this action down to the heel, so that the whole sole is covered.

3 When your thumbs reach the heel, release the pressure and glide both thumbs up the sides of the foot simultaneously. Then, with thumbs touching at the tips, draw them down the foot with a firm, confident stroke to the heel.

4 Glide your thumbs back to the starting position and repeat the sequence four times.

• *Encourage your massage partner to enjoy the tingling sensation in their foot as the blood circulation improves.*

SOLE STRETCH

This is a stretching and releasing movement, which complements the previous movements on the sole and helps loosen and soften the foot.

1 Rest the flat of one hand on the top of your massage partner's foot. Make a loose fist with your free hand and place your knuckles just under the ball of the foot. Stroke your fist firmly down the sole of the foot toward the heel so that the backs of your fingers, not your knuckles, press into the skin. This creates a deep and very satisfying stretch. Repeat three times.

2 Now use the heel of your free hand to make a firm, circular movement around the arch of the foot. Make a generous circle maintaining as much contact as possible. Keep your hand soft and relaxed with your palm flat against the skin. Repeat three times.

STROKING THE TOP OF THE FOOT

This is a light stroking movement that can be refreshing or very calming – depending on the speed of the stroke. For best effect, you should be in a position where you can lean slightly backward. Keep your back straight and bring your elbows out to the sides.

1 Hold your massage partner's foot with both hands, your thumbs resting underneath and the tips of all fingers placed in a line on the top of the toes. Lift your elbows to the sides to stroke all eight fingers lightly down the top of the foot to the ankle.

2 Stroke your fingers around the ankle bone – your right hand on the right side, and left hand on the left side – in a circular movement.

3 Now lean back and, at the same time, bring your fingers back up to the toes with an even lighter pressure than before.

4 Repeat this sequence four times.

• *Be careful not to press too hard on the bones on the top of the foot – check your pressure with your massage partner.*

TOE TONIC

This movement has a surprisingly relaxing effect. Move your elbows out to the sides to do it more effectively.

1 Hold the foot in both hands, fingers overlapping on the sole of the foot and thumbs on top. Place your thumbs on the base line of the toes between the big toe and second toe. Now stroke the pad of one thumb downward with a fairly firm pressure for about an inch (2.5cm). Your thumb follows the groove between the tendons on the top of the foot. As one thumb completes a stroke, the other follows the same path in a rhythmical way.

2 Repeat this wave-like movement, one thumb flowing after the other, for around 10 strokes.

3 Move your hands to repeat this movement along the other groves on the top of the foot, finishing with the little toe.

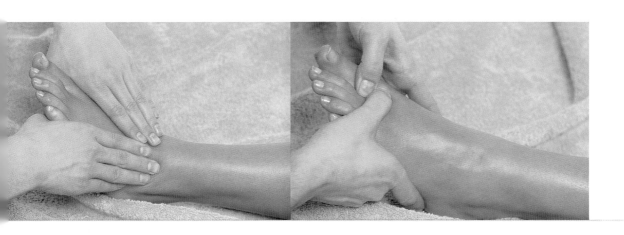

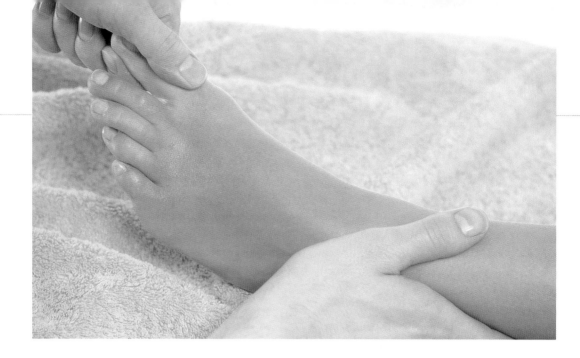

TOE SQUEEZING AND STRETCHING

This sequence is refreshing and reviving for tired feet. It helps mobilize stiff joints, strengthens muscles and stimulates the blood circulation, bringing warmth, nourishment and relaxation. Do not try to reshape malformed toes – work around them. Avoid this movement if your partner has painful, swollen or arthritic joints. Move your position and change working hands as necessary as it can be rather fiddly with small toes. You may find it helpful to lift your elbows out to the sides.

1 Hold the foot with one hand. Use the other hand to grasp your massage partner's big toe between your thumb and index finger. Hold the toe at the base, not the tip, ensuring it is well supported. Now rotate the toe slowly and deliberately in a clockwise direction three times. Then rotate it in the other direction three times. Keep the movement smooth and continuous but always work within your partner's range of movement. Do not force the action.

2 With your thumb and index finger held in the same position, gently roll and squeeze the toe as you move your hand toward the tip.

3 Glide your thumb and index finger back to the starting position and then gently pull them toward you so they slide along the length of the toe to achieve a pleasant, stretching sensation. Gradually allow them to float off the end of the toes. To create a really relaxing effect, continue the movement as though pulling a piece of string from the tips of the toes.

4 Repeat this sequence of movements on each toe in turn finishing with the little toe.

• *You may find it easier to rotate all five toes together.*

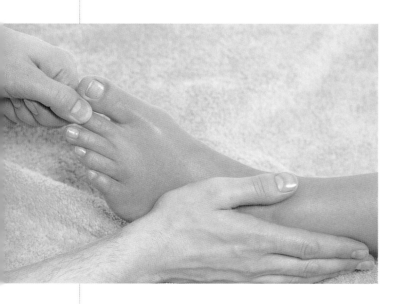

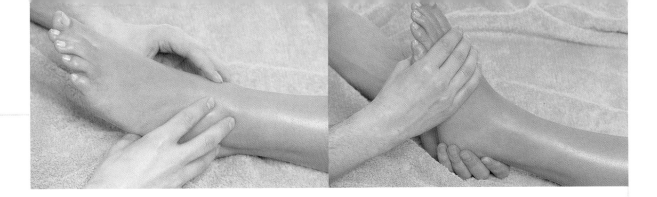

ANKLE KNEADING

This movement helps to refresh and relax stiff, tired and puffy ankles by squeezing out waste products and excess fluid, and encouraging a healthy supply of blood to nourish the surrounding tissues.

1 Clasp the foot so the heel is cupped in both hands. Place your fingers around the ankle bone and thumbs on the arch (do not press with the thumbs, simply allow them to rest on the skin). Use the fleshy pads of two or more fingers to make small circular kneading movements around the two rounded prominences on either side of the ankle. Massage both sides of the ankle simultaneously. Repeat three times.

2 Now cup the heel of the foot in the palm of one hand. With your hand still held in this cupped position, use the palm and fingers to gently massage your partner's heel with a firm circular action.

3 Release your cupped hand to enable you to massage the Achilles tendon at the back of the heel, between your thumb and fingers. Use a circular motion working up both sides of the Achilles tendon toward the back of the calf. Keep the pressure light and comforting.

• *Use your free hand to offer support to the foot.*

ANKLE ROTATING

This simple rotation movement helps ease the tendons and ligaments around the ankle joints and stretches and relaxes the Achilles tendon. Ankle rotations are also beneficial for improving blood circulation to cold feet, and preventing puffy ankles. If your massage partner has fragile bones or painful, swollen or arthritic ankles, check with her doctor that this movement is appropriate. Work within your massage partner's range of movement. Do not force the foot into an uncomfortable position.

1 Place one hand in a cupped position to support the heel of the foot. Use the other hand to gently hold the foot at the base of the toes and then rotate it from the ankle in a clockwise direction three times. Repeat the movement rotating the foot in the other direction.

2 With hands in the same position, stretch the top of the foot toward you. Hold and release. Then push it away from you in a slow, controlled and rhythmical movement. Hold and release. Repeat around five times.

• *When practised regularly ankle rotations can make a real difference to flexibility and circulation.*

FINAL TOUCH

Complete your foot massage with some very gentle strokes to calm and soothe the sensory nerve endings and bring a feeling of deep peace and relaxation.

1 Use both hands to make soft strokes with the tips of your fingers over the whole of the foot. Make the movement slow but definite. Work from the ankle to the toes. Repeat three times.

2 Gradually decrease the pressure so that your fingers hardly touch the skin in a feather-like movement. Allow your hands to slide very slowly off the end of the toes. Repeat three times.

3 Hold the foot securely between your palms for a few seconds.

Everyone can benefit from hand and foot
massage – from the very young to the very old
– not only physically but emotionally too. And
those benefits are even greater when the
massage is given with love and tenderness by
a family member or close friend.

7 Massage
for all ages

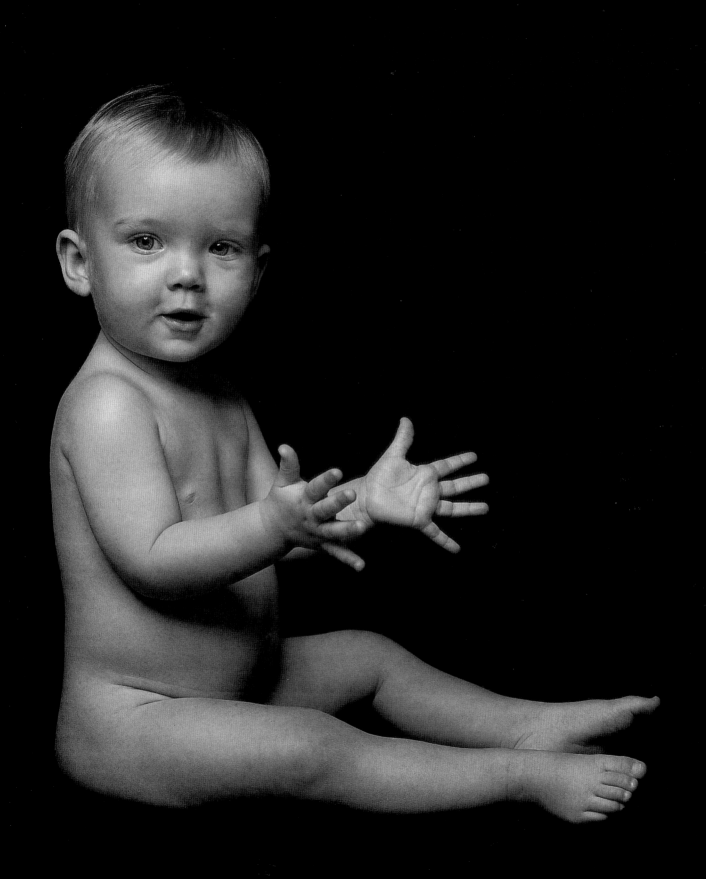

Massage during pregnancy

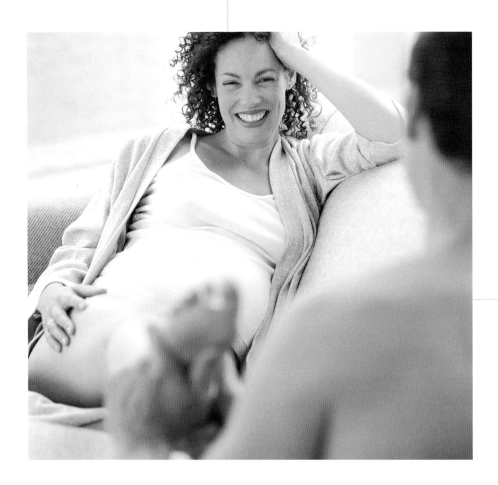

T he benefits of massage during pregnancy and childbirth are now so well recognized that many nurses and midwives are learning the techniques and actively
encouraging partners to develop their own massage skills. Pregnancy brings
increased demands on mind, body and spirit and many women find themselves
riding a roller-coaster of emotional and physical ups and downs. A gentle hand or foot massage, or indeed, a manicure or pedicure, can help during this exciting but stressful time.

Follow the routines on previous pages using plenty of light, calming massage strokes. Avoid any deep or vigorous movements during pregnancy. Choose a good quality nourishing cream or oil but do not add any essential oils without the advice of a qualified clinical aromatherapist.

Benefits for mothers-to-be

- Simple hand or foot massage can ease ante-natal anxieties and encourage deep relaxation in preparation for a more positive childbirth experience.
- Massage allows time to unwind and recharge, so increasing energy levels and making it easier to cope with the exhausting physical stresses of pregnancy.
- Nourishing creams and oils help moisturize skin and cuticles, which often become extremely dry during pregnancy.
- Foot massage can release tension in tired feet and help prevent swollen ankles so often associated with pregnancy.
- Massage releases chemicals known as endorphins, which are the body's natural painkillers, and sends them racing around the body to help boost well-being and alleviate general aches and pains.
- Manicure and pedicure help boost confidence and make you feel better about your appearance. And when you cannot reach to cut your toenails, you can rely on someone to clip them for you.
- Massage from a birth partner can be wonderfully reassuring and comforting during labour and childbirth. Although many women do not like having their bodies touched during contractions, a hand massage can help relieve tension and pain.

fact

In India and Japan, massage is regarded as an essential part of a midwife's skill. Women are traditionally given a regular massage during pregnancy and, then for forty days after the birth, new mothers and their babies receive a daily massage to help them recover from the physical and emotional strain of childbirth.

note

A few cautions

- *If you have any doubts, do not give a massage during pregnancy. Seek the advice of your massage partner's doctor or midwife if she is suffering any long-term medical condition.*

- *Check your massage partner has not developed a new medical condition such as high blood pressure or gestational diabetes, both are relatively common in pregnancy.*

- *Do not use essential oils during pregnancy, unless advised by a qualified clinical aromatherapist. Pure essential oils can have a very powerful effect and should be treated with extreme caution.*

- *Avoid massaging deeply around the heel, ankle bones and Achilles tendon as reflexologists believe these areas are related to the uterus and firm massage in the area may stimulate contractions. (Never massage the abdomen during pregnancy.)*

tip

Partners get very stressed, tired and anxious too! So set time aside to share a loving massage – and show each other just how much you are valued and cared for. Make an effort to keep massaging each other after your baby is born.

Enjoying massage with your children

Babies and children love to be held, cuddled and massaged – and not only is it a comforting, loving experience but a caring touch brings positive health benefits for both parent and child. In the animal kingdom, the young are snuggled and cuddled by their mother at every opportunity. And nature obviously knows best. Studies now reveal that babies who receive the warmth and security of close physical contact in their early days tend to cry less, have fewer tantrums and sleep more soundly. Similarly, parents can benefit from nurturing their children with touch. Research among new mothers shows that giving regular massage to their babies helps boost confidence, promote well-being and ease the baby-blues.

Sharing the caring

Expressing love and affection through touch is a basic parental instinct. Most parents naturally enjoy playing games of "Round and Round the Garden" or "This Little Piggy" with their child's tiny hands and feet. And as children get older, it is instinctive for parents to rub a sore spot to ease aches and pains, or offer comforting strokes to soothe and reassure. The physical and emotional benefits of the therapeutic power of touch can be extended still further by giving your child a regular hand and foot massage – whatever her age – whenever you feel she needs some extra love and attention.

Children enjoy giving massage, too. Young people have fewer inhibitions about touch and find it perfectly natural to communicate love for parents, siblings and friends through their hands. Indeed, you may well find that your child has a wonderfully firm and caring touch that brings almost instant benefits of relaxation and well-being – to both giver and receiver. Hand and foot massage can also be beneficial during those stormy teenage years when many parents and adolescents seem to be at loggerheads. Current studies show that the "warring sides" still hold a great affection for each other – they just do not always know how to show it. A caring hand or foot massage can go some way toward keeping open the channels of communication.

Giving and receiving

As hands and feet are so accessible, you can massage them anywhere, at anytime. And there is no need to undress, which appeals to many children, teenagers and adults. There is no need to make it a formal session or follow the steps rigidly, just take advantage of any opportunity when you are both in the mood for massage.

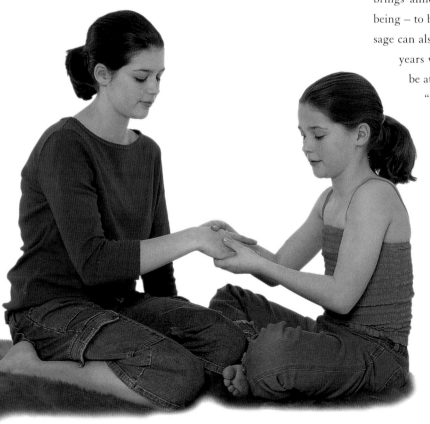

All children are different and you will soon start to discover their particular likes and dislikes, skills and preferences. Indeed, getting to know your child's character and changing moods is one of the pleasures of sharing a massage with each other. Do not force your child either to give or receive a massage; judge the right time. And stop as soon as either of you becomes bored or grumpy. Try again another time.

The following routine provides a few suggestions for a quick and simple hand and foot massage to share with your child. You can follow the whole sequence or massage hands and feet at different times. Chances are that once you have massaged your child a few times, she will be keen to return the favour and also to massage friends and siblings. However, it may be best that she does not use oil, as you could both get rather messy!

Massaging your child safely

- Choose your massage oil with care as a child's skin is very sensitive – make sure it is suitable. Avoid nut oils and all pure essential oils unless advised by a qualified clinical aromatherapist.
- Do not use oil on young children's hands in case they rub it in their eyes.
- Always get the go-ahead from the midwife or health visitor before massaging a baby.
- Do not massage if the child is unwell, particularly if he or she has a fever or is being given medication. Wait at least one week after immunization.
- Work carefully around any areas of broken skin – but avoid massage if your child has a rash or skin infection.
- Massage movements should be light and gentle using soft, flowing strokes that glide over the surface of the skin.

Get cosy

Position yourself so you have as much close contact with your child as possible. You both need to be comfortable and well-supported so you can move freely and breathe easily. Check that you do not need to twist or stretch.

- A baby will love the security and warmth of your lap. Sit on a cushion with your back supported, if possible, against a wall or heavy piece of furniture. Try cushions of different sizes to find the most comfortable one for you. Place the baby on your lap, with your legs crossed or together and knees bent. Rest her on a changing mat, cushion or pillow covered in a towel.
- If you suffer from back pain, try resting the baby on a table or changing unit that is the correct height . Never leave a baby unattended on a table or other high position.
- For a young child, try sitting with your legs stretched out in front of you in a V shape with the baby lying on the floor between your legs.
- An older child or adolescent may enjoy being massaged in a favourite chair, sofa or bed or whilst sitting on the floor. Rest hands or feet on a towel-covered pillow so they can be reached comfortably while maintaining eye-to-eye contact.

checklist

Things you will need:

- *Pillow, cushion or changing mat. Cover with a clean, soft, warm towel.*
- *Good quality oil or cream suitable for a baby or child's delicate skin (only needed for foot massage). Ask your pharmacist for advice.*
- *Wooden or plastic spatula for cream.*
- *Spare towel and baby wipes.*

Things to do:

- *Ensure the room is warm and free from draughts.*
- *Remove jewellery that may scratch the child's skin.*
- *Check that your nails are short, smooth and clean.*
- *Wash your hands in warm water.*
- *Check that you are both in a comfortable position.*

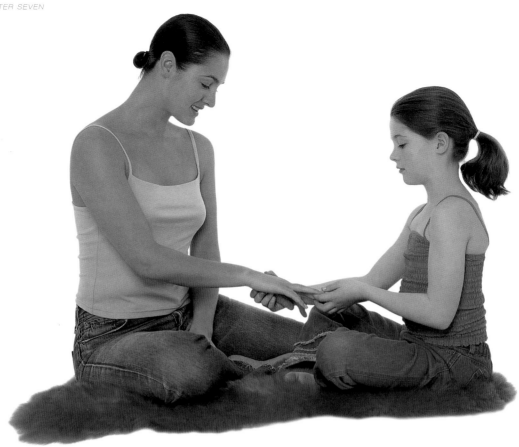

Foot massage

Place a tiny drop (half the size of a 5p coin) of suitable oil or cream in the palm of one hand. Rub your hands together briskly so they are warm.

Saying hello

Hold the child's feet securely, one in each hand, with fingers on top and thumbs beneath. Enjoy the softness of the child's skin against your skin. Keep the touch gentle but confident. Hold for a minute or so to help him or her feel reassured in your presence. Slowly remove your hands in a stroking action from ankle to toe.

• *Repeat these soothing strokes if children appear fractious to help them relax and prevent the movements causing tickles.*

note

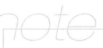

Your child is very receptive to your moods, so try to stay as calm, relaxed and confident as possible. Allow plenty of time so your child has your full attention. If you feel stressed or rushed, leave the massage until another time.

Sole strokes

With hands cradling the baby's feet, gently massage the soles of the feet with the fleshy pads of your thumbs. Move your thumbs in circles using a very light, even pressure so that they glide over the top of the skin. Mould your hands to the shape of the baby's delicate feet.

• *If feet feel ticklish try making the movements just a little deeper.*

Foot rub

Sandwich your child's right foot between your palms. Keeping your hands soft, move the flat of your hands gently backward and forward across the top and bottom of the foot. Repeat on the left foot.

• *This is a lovely way of warming cold feet.*

Toe squeeze

Cup your right hand under the heel of the child's right foot to offer support. Using the thumb and forefinger of your free hand, softly squeeze and then pull the big toe very, very gently, allowing your hand to float from the tip in a gentle, stretching action. Do not tug the toe. Repeat on each toe in turn, finishing with the little toe. Repeat the sequence on the left foot.

tip

If you have enjoyed sharing hand and foot massage with your baby, ask your health visitor to recommend a parent and baby massage class in your area. You will meet other parents and learn how to give your child a full body massage, with an expert on hand to guide you.

tip

As you massage your baby's feet, let the infant's hands explore your body too. But, as tiny hands tend to enjoy stroking your face and rearranging your hair, do take off your glasses first!

Foot hold

Complete the foot massage sequence by holding your child's feet in the warmth of your hands. Hold for a minute or so as you breathe deeply and evenly.

• *Cover your child's feet with a towel so they stay warm while you are massaging the child's hands.*

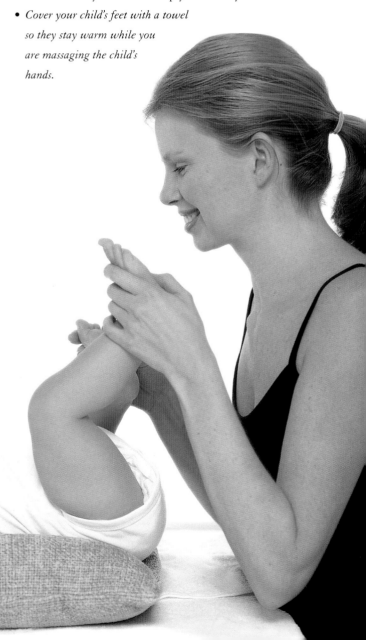

Hand massage

Greeting the hands

If you have any oil or cream on your hands use a baby wipe or towel to remove any excess and avoid the risk of babies rubbing their eyes with oily hands. Hold your child's hands gently in yours for a minute or so.

- *A child will enjoy the reassuring sound of your voice so softly talk, hum or sing.*

Palm circles

Hold your child's right hand, palm facing upward, with one hand on either side. Your fingers rest on the back of the hand and thumbs in the palm. Gently uncurl her hand, and using the fleshy pads of your thumbs, make small circles round the palm and up the backs of her fingers and thumb. Keep the pressure very light and even so the strokes skim over her skin. Repeat on her left hand.

Finger circles

Hold and support your child's right wrist in one hand. Using the index finger and thumb of your free hand, gently squeeze and rotate the thumb on her right hand. Repeat on each finger in turn, finishing with the little finger. Repeat the sequence on the left hand.

- *Be extremely gentle, do not force the action.*

Finger stroking

With your child's right hand supported at the wrist, use the fleshy pads of the fingertips on your free hand to gently stroke along the top of the hand from the wrist to the finger tips. Your touch should be featherlike as your fingers float slowly off the end of her fingertips. Do around 10 of these light strokes. Repeat on the left hand.

Signalling the end

Conclude by holding your child's hands in the same way as the start of the massage. This brings the massage to an end in a calm and balanced way.

Massage and the older generation

The warmth of the human touch through massage can be especially valuable for older people. Massage is a way of showing your respect and affection for older relatives and friends in a way that words cannot always express. Increasingly, nurses are also realizing the physical and psychological benefits of "professional love" and learning massage skills to support medical practice in the care of patients in hospitals, hospices and residential homes. Gentle hand and foot massage is particularly beneficial for less mobile elderly people as there is no need to change position.

Easing aches and pains

On a physical level, receiving a regular hand or foot massage combined with hand and foot mobility exercises can help strengthen muscles and keep joints flexible and mobile. This is important as we get older as it enables us to enjoy a better quality of life and continue participating in favourite activities or pastimes. Massage also boosts blood and lymph circulation and keeps skin soft and supple, thus helping to prevent many of the hand and foot problems associated with ageing. It also gives a caring friend or relative the chance to check the health and conditions of elderly hands or feet so any disorders (see page 46) can be treated at an early stage. Everyone in their later years should be encouraged to examine their own feet regularly using a mirror.

Boosting self-esteem

Many older people can find themselves alone at the end of their lives when they may have spent a life giving love to others. There may no longer be people there to hug or kiss them goodbye and hello. Receiving a massage can bring a caring touch back into an older person's life and go some way toward alleviating any feelings of isolation and loneliness. The tenderness of someone else's touch can boost self-esteem and promote optimism and well-being.

Growing older brings a whole new set of fears and worries – research shows that a simple five-minute hand or foot massage can reduce anxiety levels and relieve emotional stress. A gentle massage aids relaxation and brings an inner calm, which can help make it just that little bit easier to cope with a difficult situation.

Massage with care

Most older people will gain great pleasure and benefit from a hand or foot massage. However, it important to be sensitive to your partner's emotional and physical state of health. Always ask her permission and stop if she shows any signs of tiredness or distress. You should be aware that your touch may trigger an expression of sorrow or sadness. Be prepared to listen. Do not expect to be able to answer difficult questions, but just by paying attention you are providing great emotional comfort.

Ensure your massage partner is in a comfortable position and can move and breathe freely during the massage. Keep the massage light and short, and modify your movements to suit her particular needs. Use plenty of soothing feathering strokes and reassuring holds. Simply holding your massage partner's hand or foot in the warmth of your palms for a few minutes can generate

warmth, increase circulation and reduce stiffness.

As we get older our joints tend to become stiff, painful and swollen. Massage can be very soothing but should always be performed with great care around affected joints. Never work directly over a hot, swollen or inflamed joint as massage creates heat that can aggravate the condition. Apply gentle massage above and below the joint to improve blood circulation and remove excess waste products and fluid from the area. Stroke from the toes up to the ankles, and from the fingers to the wrists. Finish with a few gentle mobility exercises (see page 116) but never force the movement.

With age the skin often becomes thin, dry or fragile and can be easily damaged – so keep your pressure light with plenty of long, sweeping strokes. Ensure your nails are short and remove any rings or jewellery that could scratch the skin. Another condition associated with ageing is osteoporosis, which causes bones to lose their density and become weak and brittle. Avoid strong pressure on delicate bones as this could cause a fracture. Be especially careful of the fragile bones in the wrists. Keep your touch light, gentle and comforting.

Manicure and pedicure treatments are not simply cosmetic luxuries – they are valuable conditioning therapies for hands and feet.

Giving a
manicure
and pedicure

A good manicure or pedicure includes a relaxing massage, which can stimulate local blood circulation, strengthen nails, improve skin condition and offer protection from daily wear and tear.

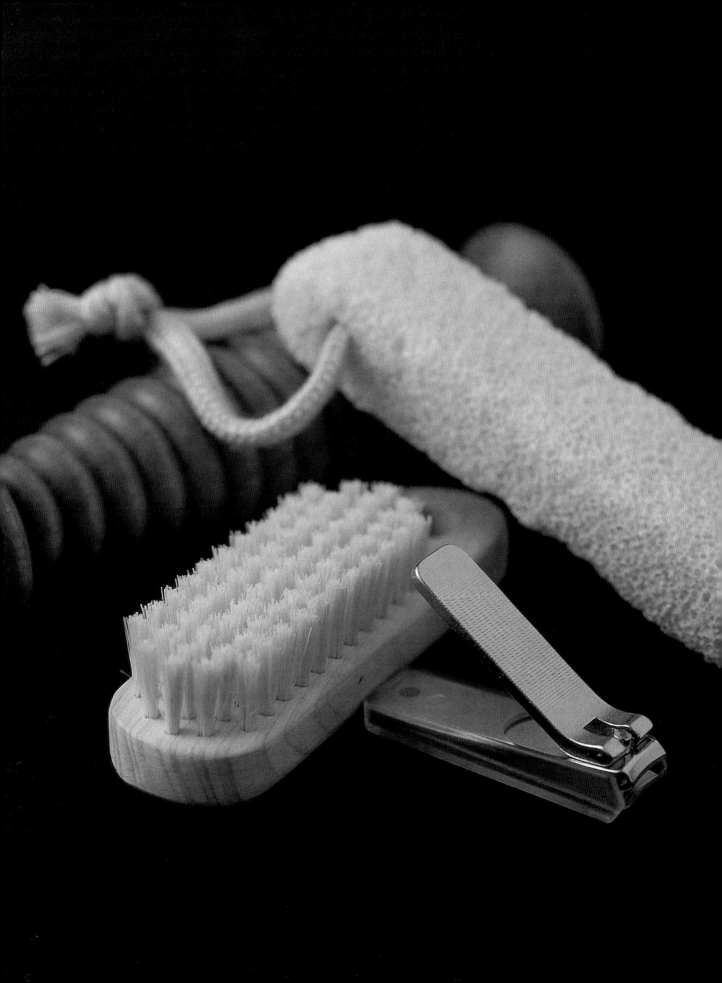

Giving a manicure

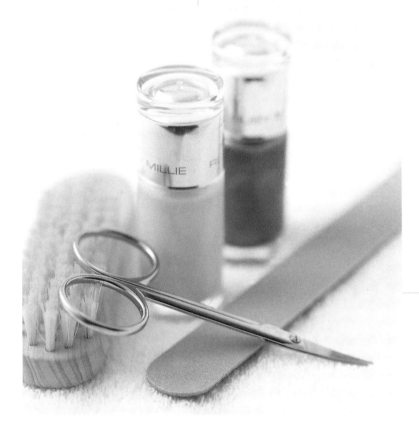

S et half an hour aside and treat a friend or relative to a quick and easy manicure or pedicure. The following steps can easily be adapted for a do-it-yourself treatment, too. Taking time and trouble to care for your hands is a great morale-booster. It is no coincidence that patients in hospital report a greater sense of relaxation and well-being when they have had their hands manicured by a Red Cross volunteer. You will find hands respond quickly to some care and attention.

checklist
Things you will need

- Three small towels – for drying hands and placing over the table.
- Paper towels – to absorb any spillage and catch nail clippings or filings.
- Cotton wool balls – for removing polish and placing on tips of orange sticks. Choose natural cotton wool as it is better at absorbing polish and less likely to stick to nails.
- Cologne (optional) – for cleaning hands.
- Nail enamel remover – for removing old polish. Use sparingly and choose a good quality acetone-free moisturizing remover as this will not cause brittle-ness and dryness.
- Nail scissors (optional) – for cutting long nails.
- Emery board – for filing nails. Avoid metal nail files as they can tear or split your nails. Emery boards usually have different textures on each side. The coarser side is used to take off excess length and the smoother, finer side for shaping the nail and removing any rough edges or snags. If the nails are weak, only use the finer side.
- Hand soak – fill a small bowl half full with warm water. Add a small drop of mild shampoo as it is less drying than most soaps or washing up liquids. Alternatively, add some sweet almond oil or three drops of pure essential oil (see Chapter 3).
- Cuticle softener or sweet almond oil – for loosening tough cuticles.
- Natural bristle nail brush – for scrubbing nails.
- Hoof stick, or orange stick tipped with cotton wool, for gently pushing back the cuticles and cleaning under the nails. Do not use anything metal and steer clear of cuticle knives, which take skill to use properly. It is important not to cut the cuticle as it offers protection and prevents foreign bodies getting beneath the skin – if the skin is damaged this could lead to a nail infection.
- Suitable cream or oil – for massaging into the skin. Take a look at Chapter Three to help make a selection.
- Wooden or plastic spatula – for applying cream.
- Nail buffer – for boosting blood circulation and polishing nails to a natural shine.
- Buffing paste (optional) – for adding an extra shine to nails.
- Basecoat and nail enamel (optional) – always use a clear basecoat to give a smoother surface and prevent enamel discolouring nails.

checklist
Things to do

- Lay out your tools so that everything is to hand.
- Remove any jewellery from yourself and the recipient of the treatment. (Keep it nearby so it does not get left behind.)
- Wash and warm your hands. Cover any cuts or abrasions with sticking plaster.
- Ask your partner to:
  – wear old clothes (or offer an apron or similar to cover her clothing and protect from any accidental spillage) and roll sleeves up to the elbow;
  – wash or cleanse hands with wipes or cotton wool soaked in cologne.

Working in comfort

You should both be sitting at the correct height and close enough so you do not need to lean forward. One of the most practical positions is to sit facing each other across a small table. Spread a towel over the table, then fold another towel into a pad as a support for your partner's elbow. Put a paper towel in place to collect any nail filings for quick and easy disposal. Keep the third towel by your side to use as necessary. An alternative position is to sit opposite each other with a towel-covered pillow on your lap.

Plan your manicure

Before you begin, examine your partner's hands thoroughly to get a feel for them. Check that she is not suffering from an infectious nail or skin disease as it would be unwise to continue with a manicure, or that she has any conditions where special care should be taken with the massage step (see page 46). You also need to find out if she has any allergies to creams, oils or nail cosmetics. If she is allergic to nail enamel, then leave out the final step of the manicure. Ask about personal preferences too, such as nail shape and enamel colour.

Take the opportunity to look at the general condition of your partner's nails and skin – you may like to offer some of the advice on hand care outlined in Chapter Nine.

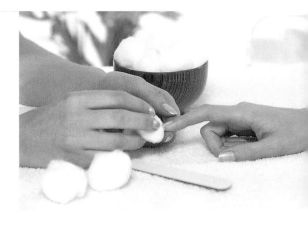

REMOVE OLD ENAMEL

This step ensures that all traces of old polish are removed allowing you to begin afresh.

Soak a cotton pad or ball with nail enamel remover and press on the nail for a moment, then wipe off slowly. A quick swipe is not enough to dissolve polish, especially glittery textures. If necessary, use a tipped orange stick soaked in nail enamel remover to clean up the cuticle and free edge of the nail.

Treat yourself to a professional manicure to keep your hands or nails in good condition. Watch the expert at work and learn. Do not worry if your nails are bitten or battered – the manicurist has seen plenty of similar hands and will have helpful advice to offer. And once you see how much better your nails look after a manicure, you will feel more inclined to look after them.

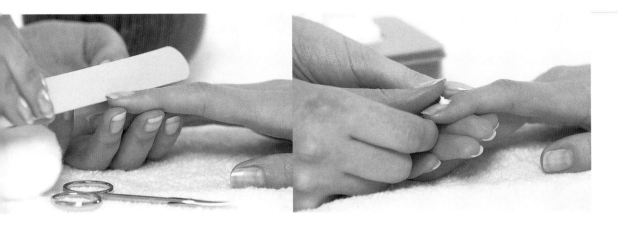

FILE THE NAILS

Now shape the nails. Your partner may have a strong view on this. If not, file the tips to the same shape as the base of the nail. Begin by doing this step and the next step on the right hand first.

Shape each nail in turn with the emery board. A good guide to correct filing technique is to hold the emery board as though about to shake hands with it. Tilt the emery board at a 45° angle so that you concentrate on the underside of the nail. Use the finer, smoother side of the emery board to file the free edge, working from the side to the centre to form a gentle curve. Work in one direction only with long, rhythmical strokes. Avoid a sawing action on one spot, which can cause the nail layers to split. Be careful not to file deep into the nail corners as this weakens the edge and the nail is more likely to split.

• *If the nails are very long it is quicker to trim them to the approximate length with nail scissors first. Cut from one side to the centre, and repeat on the other side.*

SOFTENING THE CUTICLES

This step helps soften and loosen cuticles (the dead skin around the edge of the nails) so they can be more easily pushed back.

Using the tip of your index finger, massage a small amount of cuticle cream or almond oil into each nail base and the surrounding skin on the fingers.

• *If cuticles are very dry and hard, soak fingernails in a small bowl of warm almond oil for five minutes and then massage the oil into the cuticles.*

SOAK THE NAILS

This step helps to loosen any stubborn dirt from around the nails and helps soften cuticles.

Place the right hand into a hand soak. Leave in the bowl for around three to five minutes. While the right hand is soaking, repeat the previous two steps on the left hand. Then place the left hand in the hand soak (see page 101).

• *Try putting some coloured pebbles in the bowl so your partner can play with them while her nails are soaking.*

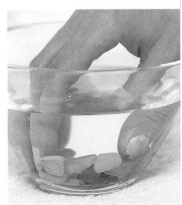

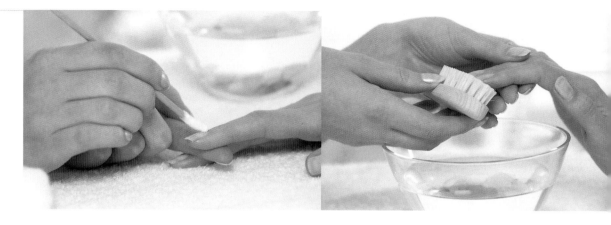

PUSH BACK THE CUTICLES

This helps improve the appearance of the cuticle area and pre-vents cuticles from attaching to the nail plate, which could cause the cuticle to split.

1 Take the right hand from the water and pat each nail and finger dry with a towel. Apply a little cuticle cream to the nail base of the fingers and massage it in gently.

2 The cuticles should now be soft enough for you to gently ease them back using a hoof stick, or orange stick tipped with cotton wool. For best effect, hold the hoof stick, or orange stick, like a pen. Be gentle, do not apply too much pressure. Repeat on the left hand.

• Alternatively, wrap a soft towel around your fingertip and use this to gently push back the cuticles. You can do this on your own cuticles after a bath.

WASH THE HANDS

This step helps remove any excess cuticle cream, which is caustic and could dry or burn the skin.

Dip both hands in the warm hand soak to wash off any remaining cuticle remover. Then take hands from the bowl and pat dry. If your partner's hands or nails are a little dirty, use a soft, natural bristle nail-brush to scrub away any dirt or stains. The light, rubbing action helps increase blood circulation to the nails so encouraging healthy growth.

MASSAGE THE HANDS AND ARMS

This feels wonderful! It also helps boost the circulation, improve joint mobility, nourish dry skin and relax your partner.

Apply a rich moisturizing cream or oil to your hands. Rub your hands together so they are warm and well lubricated. Now follow the steps in the routine in Chapter Five. At the end of the massage, ensure that all the cream or oil has been massaged in or remove any excess with tissue. You could also dip your partner's fingertips in the warm water and scrub the nails gently with a nail brush. Any stubborn dirt can be removed with an orange stick – but do not dig too deep as this will pull the nail from the nail bed.

• Massage cream or oil into the nail bases to help keep cuticles soft and ensure nails are well hydrated.

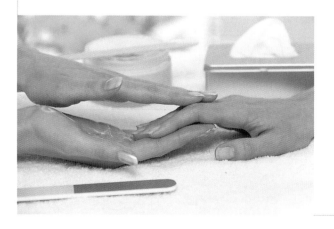

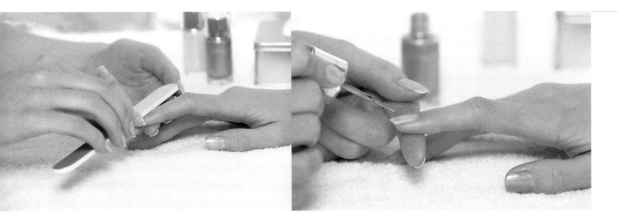

BUFF THE NAILS

Buffing is a simple technique that brings quick results. It gives the nail plate a natural, healthy shine, helps smooth out ridges and also stimulates the blood supply so promoting healthier, stronger nails. Buffing is also useful for removing yellowish tints on the nails caused by nicotine or sunlight.

With the buffer held loosely in your hand, work on each nail plate in turn. Buff in one direction only from the base of the nail to the free edge. Use firm, smooth strokes. Around six strokes for each nail is usually sufficient – do not overdo it. Tidy up nails with an emery board to give a smooth finish.

● *If you are not using nail enamel, apply a small amount of buffing paste to achieve an extra shine.*

tip

Men benefit from manicures too – and usually thoroughly enjoy the pampering. The only real differences are that most men prefer to have nails cut straight across and not shaped at the sides and that their nails may take a bit more effort to scrub clean. It is unlikely that a man would want nail enamel but buffing can give his nails a healthy sheen.

APPLY NAIL ENAMEL

This is a personal choice. Offer your partner a selection of colours before applying.

1 First make sure that the nail is free from any grease or cream as this will cause the enamel to bubble or go streaky. Apply a clear base coat and leave to dry for 15 minutes. Avoid waving your hands to dry them as this may create an uneven texture.

2 When the base coat is completely dry, apply varnish in three straight strokes – one down the middle, and one on each side. Remove any enamel on surrounding skin with an orange stick tipped with cotton wool. Allow to dry thoroughly before using hands.

● *Before using nail polish, roll the bottle in the palms of your hands. Avoid shaking it as this creates air bubbles, which can lead to chipping.*

Giving a pedicure

Regular foot care including a pedicure and foot massage not only helps make feet look more attractive but also reduces hard skin, odours and sweat, relaxes tired, aching feet and helps prevent many common problems from developing.

Check your position

It is worth spending a little time and effort making sure that you are both comfortable and at the correct height. One of the most practical positions is sitting facing each other. Place a small table between you with a towel-covered cushion to support your partner's leg and foot. Ensure that the knee is slightly bent so the foot is relaxed. The foot bowl can be placed on a towel on the floor. Keep a towel handy for drying your partner's feet, and another for wrapping them to keep warm.

checklist
Things to do

- Check your partner has no infectious or contagious skin or nail diseases that would make it unwise to continue with the pedicure, and that she does not have any conditions where special care should be taken with the massage step (see page 120). Ask about allergies to creams or oils. Discuss choice of nail enamel colour.
- Lay out everything you need so that it is all to hand.
- Ask your partner to wear loose clothing and remove shoes, tights and socks. Trousers should be rolled up to the knees.
- Remove your jewellery and your partner's toe rings or anklets.
- Wash your hands. Cover any cuts or abrasions with sticking plaster.

checklist
Things you will need

- Three towels – for drying feet and warming feet.
- Cotton wool balls – to remove polish and place on top of orange sticks. Choose natural cotton wool as it is better at absorbing polish and less likely to stick to nails.
- Paper towels – to absorb any spillage and catch nail clippings.
- Nail enamel remover – for taking off old polish. Use sparingly and choose a good quality moisturizing remover that is free from acetone, which can cause brittleness and dryness.
- Nail clippers – for cutting nails to the right length.
- Emery board – for filing nails. Do not use metal files as these can damage nails.
- Foot soak – use a large bowl half full with warm water. The bowl should be deep enough to immerse the feet to the ankles. A washing-up bowl is ideal. Add a few drops of mild shampoo or bath lotion as it is less drying than most soaps or washing-up liquids. Alternatively, add some sweet almond oil or three drops of pure essential oil (see Chapter Three).
- Cuticle softener or sweet almond oil – for loosening tough cuticles.
- Natural bristle nail brush – for scrubbing nails.
- Hoof stick, or orange stick tipped with cotton wool, for gently pushing back the cuticles and cleaning under nails. Do not use anything metal for this job, and never use cuticle knives, which can be dangerous in untrained hands.
- Pumice stone or exfoliating cream – for removing rough skin.
- Suitable cream or oil – for massaging into the skin.
- Wooden or plastic spatula – for applying cream.
- Basecoat and nail enamel (optional) – for adding colour to the nails.

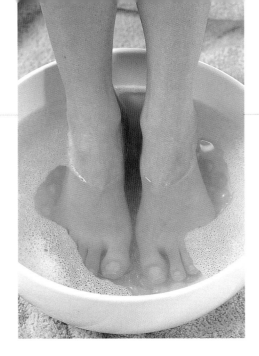

CLEANSE THE FEET

At the start of the pedicure your partner may feel concerned that her feet are smelly or dirty and otherwise unpleasant. Put her at ease by soaking her feet in a relaxing, cleansing foot soak.

1 Ask your partner to put both feet in the foot soak. Leave the feet in the bowl for three to five minutes. While her feet are soaking, encourage your partner to relax and unwind. She may like to close her eyes and enjoy the pleasing sensation of warmth on her feet.

2 Remove feet from the soak and dry thoroughly. Be extra vigilant about drying between the toes as bacteria and fungi thrive in moist, dark conditions and can cause skin disorders.

3 Soak a cotton pad with nail enamel remover and press against each nail for a few seconds, then wipe off slowly. If necessary, use a tipped orange stick soaked in nail enamel remover to clean up the cuticle and free edge of the nail.

• Use this opportunity to assess the general condition of your partner's feet and, if appropriate, offer self-care advice (see Chapter 9) for looking after her feet.

CLIP AND FILE THE NAILS

Toe nails should be kept straight, allowing only a gentle curve at the sides, as this prevents the nail cutting into the skin and so protects against ingrowing nail (see page 123). Place a tissue to collect any clippings or filings for quick disposal.

Use clippers to cut a straight line across the nail. Do not use scissors as they can split the nail. Trim the nails of the left foot in turn. Using the coarse side of the emery board, file the nails to remove any sharp corners or rough edges. Do not try to shape them or file into the corners.

• Hold the emery board so that it is slightly angled beneath the free edge of the nail. Using long strokes, file each side of the nail toward the centre.

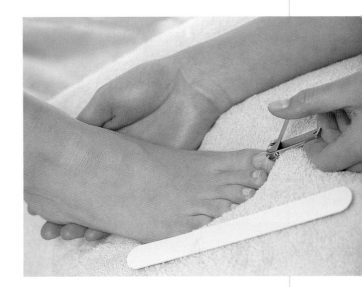

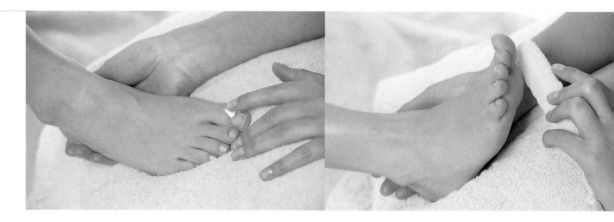

EASING BACK THE CUTICLES

This step is a must if you wish your feet to look pretty in open-toe sandals. It is also important for nail health as it keeps the cuticles in good condition.

Apply a small dab of cuticle cream or almond oil into each nail base and massage in gently with your forefinger. Now place both feet back into the warm water. Allow to soak for a minute or so. Remove and dry thoroughly. Massage a little more cuticle cream into each nail base. Ease the cuticles back very gently using a hoof stick, or orange stick tipped with cotton wool. Try using circular movements to ease the cuticle down and away from the nail. Wipe off any excess cuticle remover with cotton wool.

• *Be careful not to damage the cuticle as it acts as a protective barrier against fungi and bacteria.*

REMOVING HARD SKIN

During a pedicure, excess hard skin can be removed to improve the appearance of your partner's feet. Place some paper towel under the foot to catch any shedding skin.

If there is only a mild build-up of hard skin, massage the feet with some exfoliating cream or a mixture of damp sea salt and olive oil (about a tablespoon of each mixed to a fairly thick paste). Use a deep, circular movement, working with your fingers. On very rough, dry areas around the heels and balls of the feet, use a pumice stone, friction pad or chiropody block available from large chemists. Never use metal files or attempt to cut or shave hard skin. Avoid sawing back and forth with the pumice stone, which can be quite painful, and be careful not to over-do it as this can cause irritation.

• *If hard skin is causing pain or discomfort seek the advice of a state registered chiropodist, or podiatrist.*

tip

At last people are waking up to the need to respect our hard-working feet. There is now a wide selection of good quality natural foot care products and treatments on the market – enjoy browsing to find those that appeal to you.

note

Regular pedicures are especially important if you usually wear synthetic shoes and socks, or if you suffer from poor circulation or diabetes as it is vital to keep your feet in good condition to prevent further problems.

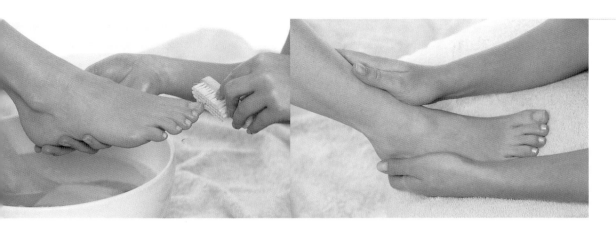

BRUSHING THE NAILS

This step helps remove any loosened dirt and all traces of cuticle remover ready for a soothing massage.

Place both feet back in the warm water. Use a natural bristle nail brush to scrub around the nails. Clean under the free edges of the nails with a cotton-tipped orange stick soaked in water. Take both feet from the water.

• At this point, remove the bowl from the working area to prevent it being knocked over.

MASSAGE THE FEET AND LEGS

Follow removal of hard skin with a moisturizing massage. This helps to relieve tension in hard working muscles and tendons and promotes general relaxation and a sense of well-being.

Apply a rich moisturizing cream or oil to your hands. Rub together so they are well lubricated. Now follow the steps in the foot massage routine in Chapter Six.

• Ensure that all the cream or oil has been massaged in, or remove any excess with tissue.

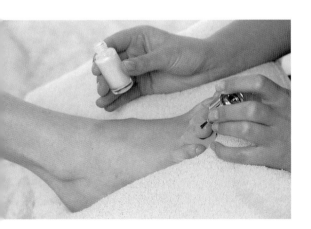

APPLY NAIL ENAMEL

Offer your partner a choice of colours – your taste may not be the same! Before applying polish, check that the nails are free from grease.

To prevent smudging, use a specially designed toe separator or divide toes with a tissue, folded lengthwise and threaded between the toes. Apply a clear base coat and leave to dry for five minutes. When the base coat is completely dry, apply varnish in three straight stokes – one down the middle, and one on each side. Clean any smudge marks with a cotton-tipped orange stick dipped in polish remover.

• Leave for 10 to 15 minutes to dry before removing toe separators. Wait at least an hour before putting on tights or shoes.

Caring for your hands and feet

Once your massage partner starts to enjoy the benefits of regular hand or foot massage, it is helpful to offer some general tips and advice to help keep skin and nails in good condition. Do not forget to follow your own advice!

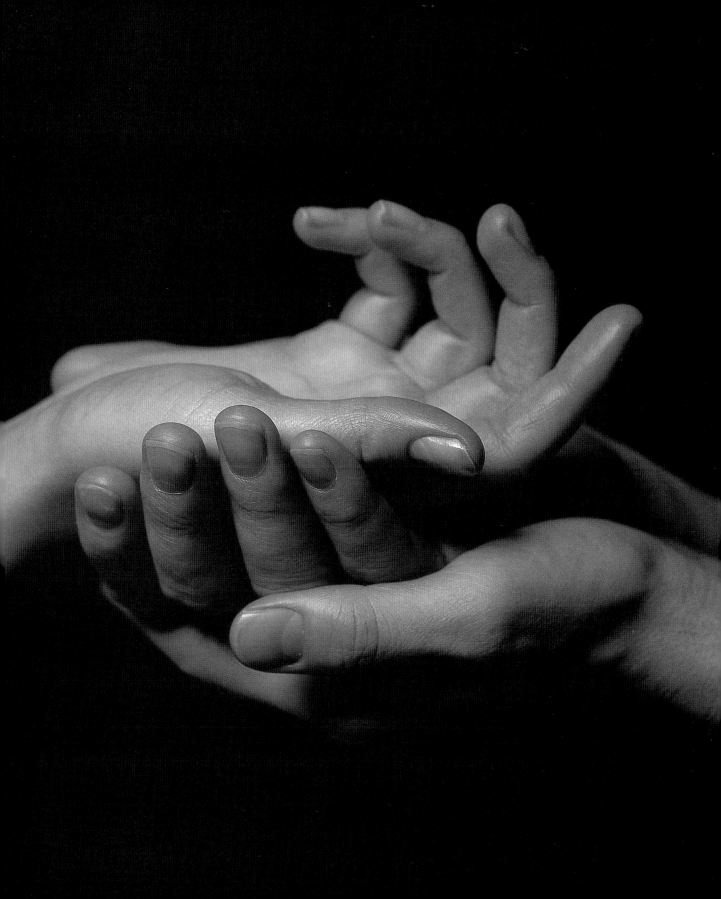

Looking after hands and feet

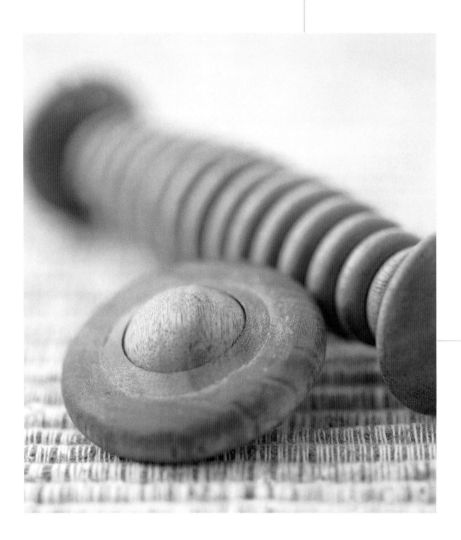

Sensible hygiene and care can enhance the benefits of massage and help prevent many common problems developing. These simple self-help measures are easy to follow and will make a noticeable difference to keeping skin and nails healthy and attractive. It is well worth spending a little time on caring for hands and feet – when they look and feel good, then you feel good too!

Clean and fresh

Wash your hands and feet every day with a gentle, soap-free cleanser. The water should be warm but not hot, which can cause drying and tightening of the skin. If you have a loss of sensation in your hands or feet, because of diabetes or other condition, check the temperature with your elbow. Rinse and dry thoroughly, especially between the toes, as bacteria and fungi thrive in warm, moist conditions. The area between the fourth and fifth toe on each foot is the most common site of infection. It is important not to share towels and flannels if a member of the family has warts, nail infection or other contagious conditions as they can be so easily passed to others. Choose shoes and socks made from natural fibres, which allow cool air to circulate. It is best not to wear the same shoes two days running; so allow shoes time to dry before wearing them again.

tip

Try massaging and rubbing one foot against the other to boost the circulation. It is amazing how dexterous your toes can be. Use the heel and sides of your feet to work into all the curves and bends to ease out all the tension and get blood flowing to the feet.

Soft and supple

Hands and feet will benefit from a relaxing soak in a bowl half full of warm water – but do not soak them for longer than five minutes as this can upset the natural balance of protective oils and has a drying effect. A handful of Dead Sea salts added to the water can help improve circulation, soften the skin and fight infection. Hard skin should be treated with care – gently rub away with a pumice stone every day to keep it under control. Attempting to remove it all in one go could lead to very sore feet. If you have a build-up of hard skin, ask the advice of a state registered chiropodist, or podiatrist.

Regular massage with a rich moisturizer will keep the skin and nails on the feet and hands supple and prevent chapping or cracking. Rub in well but avoid the area between the toes as this should be kept fairly dry to avoid infection. A useful tip is to keep pots of moisturizer in different places all over the house to jog your memory. Try this skin-softening routine: once a week, just before going to bed, apply a generous amount of moisturizing cream to your hands and feet. Now put on a pair of white cotton gloves (available at most pharmacies) and socks and allow your skin and nails to reap the benefits while you sleep.

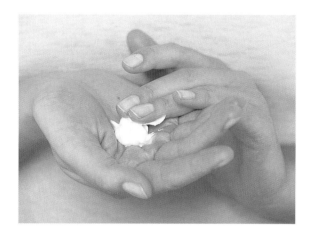

Protecting your skin

During the day it is wise to get into the habit of wearing gloves whenever your hands are immersed in water for some time – if you do not like rubber gloves then lightweight surgical gloves are suitable. Limit the amount of detergent used in washing up or cleaning. Detergent left on the skin may cause uncomfortable dryness and rashes. Always rinse your hands with fresh water after contact with detergent, especially between the fingers and under rings. Wear protective gloves for dirty, dry work such as gardening and do not forget to shield your hands from the elements: warm gloves help maintain blood circulation to the hands and nails during cold weather, or even when getting food out of the freezer.

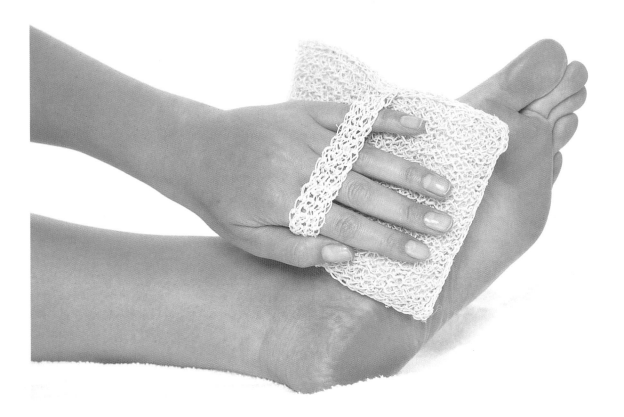

Hands also need protection from the sun's ultra-violet rays. Use a sunscreen lotion or moisturizing cream that filters out harmful rays to protect your health, and prevents dehydration and age spots – do not forget to massage sunscreen into your nails, too. Never use your nails to prize open lids or do similar jobs; find the right tool for the task or you could end up with split nails.

Early warning

It is good advice to get into the habit of inspecting your hands and feet every day – especially if you have a medical condition such as diabetes that can lead to foot disorders. Look for signs of redness, cuts, swelling or cracks in your skin, or any changes in colour or temperature. If you find it difficult to view your feet, try using a mirror, or ask a friend to look for you. If you have any doubts, then see your doctor. The earlier that problems are reported, the quicker they can be treated. Cover any breaks in the skin with a plaster to guard against infection. Keep your nails trimmed – toenails should be cut straight across. Do not pick or tear finger and toenails. They are often easier to cut after a bath, when they are softer.

Boost circulation

A sluggish blood circulation can cause misery – not only do hands and feet feel cold and uncomfortable but poor circulation is at the root of many disorders that affect the extremities. Following a few simple guidelines can help improve blood circulation but if you are concerned then see your doctor as poor circulation may be associated with a medical condition.

To boost sluggish circulation in the morning, sit on a chair or the side of a bed and move your legs briskly up and down, one after the other. The movement comes from your knees with your ankles staying soft and flexible. Then take a warm bath to pep up your circulation and raise your body temperature. Brush palms and soles with a soft body brush using firm, circular strokes. Dry thoroughly with a rough towel. Rub a moisturizing cream or oil into areas that are likely to become chilled.

After your bath, do some hand and foot mobility exercises (see page 116–9) and repeat them at regular intervals. Apparently, military guardsmen, who stand for hours on end, keep their circulation moving by wiggling their toes inside their boots!

If possible, eat breakfast and have a hot meal and plenty of hot drinks during the day to maintain body heat. Cut back on smoking as this constricts the blood vessels and makes the problem even worse. It also discolours skin and nails, and robs the body of vital nutrients. Exercise is vital to a healthy blood circulation. Walking, especially up hills, is particularly good exercise for the feet as it strengthens muscles, ligaments and tendons. Try to take a brisk walk every day, wearing correct footwear. When you get a chance to sit down – put your feet up above the level of your hips to encourage the flow of blood back to the heart.

If it is chilly outside, wrap up warm as the cold temperature hinders blood circulation to the extremities. Wear several layers of thin, loose clothing to trap body heat and put on gloves, thick socks, a scarf and hat. Avoid any clothing that restricts blood circulation – a red ring on your lower leg is a sure sign that the elastic in your socks is too tight. Try wearing thin cotton or silk socks under thick tights and choose shoes or boots with warm, inner soles. Wear bed socks at night.

Choosing footwear

Poorly fitting shoes are the cause of many foot problems. Shoes that are too narrow, tight, long, high or wide not only make feet tired and aching, but can speed up the onset of problems or aggravate existing ones.

Correct shoe fitting is not just for children. Every time you buy new shoes you should ask to have your feet measured for size and width by a trained shoe fitter. Shoe size is only a guide. Shoes that are the same size can have a different fit, depending on the style and manufacturer. The best time to buy shoes is in the afternoon as your feet tend to swell during the day. Put on both shoes and stand up and walk around.

tip

Alternate your style of footwear and heel height regularly. This helps tone up your calf muscles and reduces strain on the feet and ankles.

The shoe should be about half an inch longer than your foot with plenty of room for your toes to move. It should fit snugly at the heel and instep and be wide enough to prevent friction, squashing or rubbing when you walk. Never buy shoes in the hope that they will stretch to fit. Socks and tights should have room for some movement too. Check that there are no holes or rough edges in socks, tights or shoes.

For optimum support and comfort, choose a shoe with a heel no higher than 4 cm (1½ in) and a rounded toe. Shoes fastened by laces, straps or a buckle are preferable for foot health. Always choose the most suitable shoe for the occasion – especially sport or work. Keep high heels for special occasions as constant wear can cause muscular imbalances in the lower leg, which leads to aches and cramps. In high-heeled shoes your toes are crushed forward and the tendons on the top of the foot are stretched while the Achilles tendon at the back of the heel is shortened.

note

If your hands or feet get very cold then warm them gradually. Be wary of heating them on radiators, hot water bottles or near a fire as the sudden change in temperature can lead to further problems.

Hand
exercises

Hand and finger exercises can help boost blood circulation, ease aches and pains and maintain strength and flexibility in your hands and wrists. Repeat these exercises several times a day, and perform them as a warm-up routine just before giving a massage. It is best to remove all jewellery from your hands and wrists. You may find it more comfortable to rest your elbows on a folded towel on a table or desk for some of the exercises.

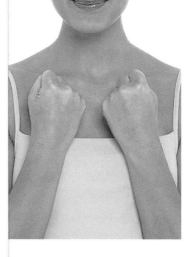

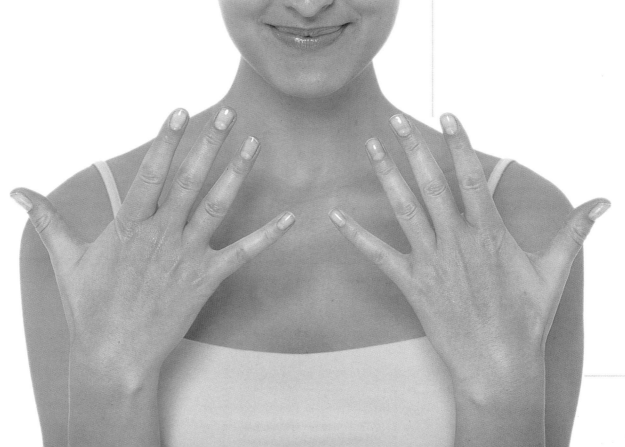

note

Hand and foot mobility exercises can be beneficial if you have arthritis, Raynaud's disease or repetitive strain injury – but if you suffer from these conditions, or any other medical condition, consult your doctor or physiotherapist before doing hand or foot exercises. It is important that all movements are tailored to your particular needs.

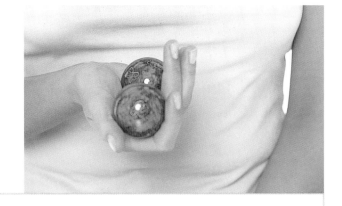

1 Make soft fists with both hands. Then quickly separate your fingers and thumbs and stretch them out as far as you can reach (see left). Hold for a count of 10. Feel the tension in your fingers. Slowly release and return to the soft fists. Repeat three times.

2 Put your hands on a flat surface with the palms facing downward. First, lift your thumbs, then each finger in turn, as though playing a piano. Return to the starting position by placing your little fingers on the surface, followed by each individual finger. Repeat three times.

3 Place the palms of your hands together in the "prayer" position. Press one hand firmly against the other and hold for a count of five. Release and repeat. With your hands in the same position, keep your wrists, thumbs and fingertips in contact while pushing out your knuckle joints to form a diamond shape with your hands (see below right). Hold for a count of five. Return to the starting position and repeat three times.

4 Try this exercise if you suffer from poor circulation in your hands. Stand with your hands by your sides. Now raise your arms in front of you as high as you can comfortably reach. Turn your wrists so that your palms face downward and then lower your arms to your sides in a swinging action. Repeat three times. Rest and repeat the sequence another three times, allowing yourself to get into a steady rhythm.

5 Hold a small soft, rubber ball (buy one specially designed for "stressbusting") or some playdough or plasticine in your hand. Squeeze and mould it in your hands to work the muscles, but without straining them. Repeat, this time holding the ball in the other hand.

6 Take a tip from the East and invest in some Chinese hand balls for a fun way to keep your hands and fingers supple (see above). These small balls, which are readily available in oriental craft shops and health food stores, work by stimulating acupuncture points on the hands to increase the flow of vital energy through the body. Hold two balls in the palm of one hand, and circle them around each other in your palm and fingers. Some even come with musical accompaniment to help soothe your nerves.

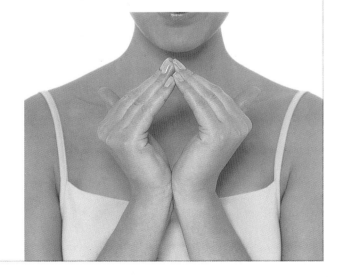

Foot *exercises*

Feet and toes need to be kept on the move. Without sufficient exercise, the muscles in your feet tend to slacken, arches weaken, joints become stiff and blood circulation slows down. These simple exercises will strengthen and relax muscles, tendons and ligaments so helping to prevent foot problems and keep your feet healthy, flexible and warm. Remove your shoes and allow your feet the chance to exercise freely – set aside a few minutes every day and you will soon notice the improvement, especially as you go up and down the stairs.

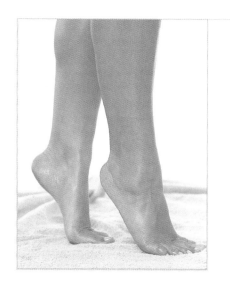

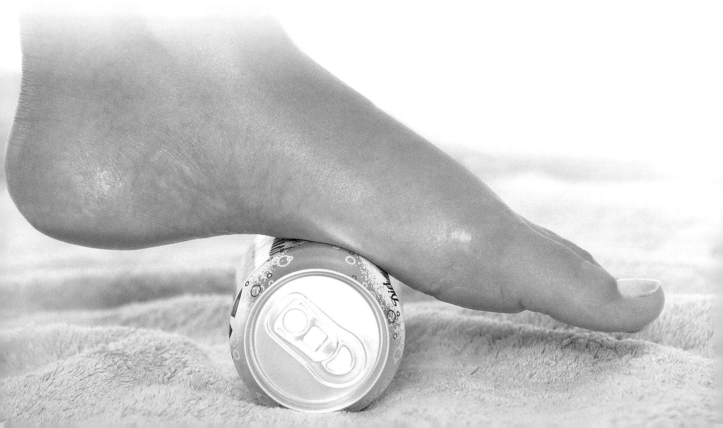

tip

1 Stand straight, feet about 20 cm (8 in) apart, toes pointing ahead. Now raise yourself up slow-ly on your toes, hold for a count of five, lower. Repeat five times. Try walking on tip toes for a few paces (see left).

2 Place a soft ball, orange or can of drink (try it cold from the fridge) under the ball of your foot and roll it backward and forward for one minute to improve circulation and relieve any aches in the arch. Repeat with the other foot. Alternatively, use a spe-cially designed foot massager (see left).

3 Sit on a chair with your feet flat on the ground. Press the toes of your left foot into the floor, and raise the toes of your right foot firmly upward. Hold for a count of three and then release slowly. Repeat with the opposite foot. This may take some practice, but do persevere. Try raising the toes individually.

4 Sitting in the same position as above, grasp a pencil with your toes. Hold for a count of five, release. Repeat. To add an extra dimension to this exercise, place a sheet of paper on the floor and try writing or drawing with the pencil.

5 Sit on the floor with your legs pointing straight ahead. Point your toes down and away from you (see below left). Hold for a count of 10. Release and repeat. Now, flex your feet so that your toes are pointing toward your nose (see below right). Hold for a count of 10. Release and repeat. Point your toes inward toward the middle of the body. Hold for a count of 10. Release and repeat. Finally move your feet out toward the side of your body. Hold for a count of 10. Release and repeat.

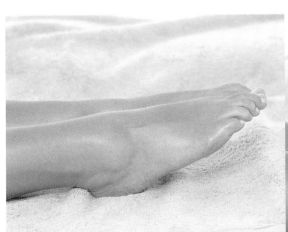 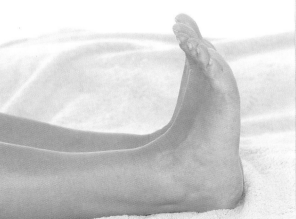

Move with grace

Good posture – whether you are walking, or sitting at a computer – helps keep feet and hands flexible and healthy, and also changes the way you look and feel. When you move with comfort and grace, you adopt an air of confidence and well-being. Walking or moving incorrectly can upset the whole balance of your body, leading to a build-up of tension in the muscles of the arms, hands, legs and feet.

When standing, picture your head balanced evenly and freely on top of your spine, with your arms and legs extending from the centre, allowing ease of movement. Lengthen and widen your spine, keeping your weight evenly distributed and shoulders relaxed and at the same height.

When driving a car, position the seat so that you are not cramped and can reach the controls with ease. Hold the steering wheel fairly loosely, with your hands resting a little lower than your shoulders. Do not grip too tightly or place your hands at the top of the steering wheel. When doing repetitive movements using your hands and fingers, take breaks every few minutes.

note

Learn to be aware of any tensions that creep into your hands and feet, legs and arms, during everyday activities. Try to make a conscious effort to relax and let go.

Common hand and foot conditions

Many people are embarrassed by hand or foot conditions – but they are extremely common, far more so than you may imagine. You can help yourself and your massage partner by learning to identify particular conditions. Although prevention is always better than cure, with early attention many of these problems can be dealt with swiftly.

Athlete's foot

This is a common fungal infection of the feet, usually affecting the skin between the toes, that affects as many as one in seven adults. It is highly contagious, and can be passed on wherever people walk barefoot, especially in moist, warm areas such as changing rooms – so wear flip-flops to avoid catching it. The first signs of athlete's foot are itchy, irritating patches of skin, especially between the fourth and fifth toes, which crack and peel, and then turn "soggy" and white, often with an unpleasant odour. The condition may also appear as rough, red, scaly skin on the soles of the feet. Treat by washing your feet daily in warm water to which you have added two drops of tea tree oil. Dry thoroughly with a clean towel, especially between the toes, and apply antifungal powder, cream or spray. Continue treatment for two weeks after it has cleared up. If the problem persists or becomes painful or irritating, see your doctor or a state registered chiropodist, or podiatrist. Avoid massage until the condition has cleared up.

Brittle nails

If a nail contains less than 12 per cent water it can become brittle and easily flake, chip, snap and split. Constant use of detergents and chemicals or immersing the hands or feet in water for long periods of time can strip the protective oils from the skin and nails so they cannot conserve moisture. Central heating, poor diet and exposing hands and feet to the elements can also be dehydrating. Nails tend to become harder and more inflexible as we get older. Treat with regular hand massage to boost blood circulation and bring nourishment to the growing nail cells. If your nails tend to be brittle, keep them short to maintain their strength. Do not try to mend split nails, but file them down with an emery board.

Bunions

These are a problem affecting the large joint at the base of the big toe causing it to protrude and push the big toe out of line so it turns toward the other toes. The skin may become red and sore, from rubbing against the side of the shoe, and the big toe joint can become swollen. The problem often runs in families, perhaps because of an inherited weakness in the joint structure, and is aggravated by wearing shoes that are too tight or narrow. It is important to wear well-fitting shoes that prevent excessive pressure on the toe. Seek professional help if a bunion becomes painful or debilitating. A state registered chiropodist, or podiatrist, can offer advice on appropriate shoes and treatment. Massage around the affected joint may be beneficial.

Callouses

These are areas of thickened skin found on the feet and hands. Patches of such hard, dry skin, which are usually caused by regular or prolonged pressure or friction, vary in size and thickness. If left untreated, callouses can become painful, and split open allowing bacteria, viruses and fungi to invade the skin. Some people have a natural tendency to form callouses because of their skin type. Elderly people are particularly prone because they tend to have less fatty tissue in their skin to act as a shock-absorber. You can control the build-up of hard skin by keeping the hands and feet clean and well moisturized. Gently rub away any patches of dry skin with a pumice stone, but don't be too vigorous. If a callous becomes painful or persists, seek the advice of your doctor or a state registered chiropodist, or podiatrist. Massage can help soften hard skin.

Chilblains

Itchy, tender, purple or pink swellings found on the extremities such as fingers, toes, ears and nose are known as chilblains. They are triggered when the superficial blood vessels go into spasm on exposure to cold. They tend to appear in winter and affect people with poor circulation. Chilblains may occur if the skin gets chilled and is then heated too rapidly by a fire, radiator or hot water bottle. Women are six times more likely to suffer than men. Chilblains can dry out, leaving cracks in the skin, which expose feet to the risk of infection. Keep your hands and feet warm and dry, and try not to scratch or rub chilblains. Regular hand and foot mobility exercises and massage using a blend of pure essential oils (see Chapter Three) can help boost circulation to unbroken chilblains. If chilblains are broken seek the advice of your doctor or (for chilblains on the feet) a state registered chiropodist, or podiatrist, on ways of promoting healing.

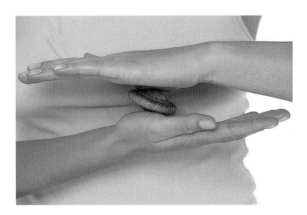

Corns

These are the most common foot problems – but they are not contagious so feet can still enjoy the benefits of massage. There are several different types of corn. Hard corns are patches of hard, yellowish skin, up to the size of a small pea, which are caused by excessive rubbing or pressure. Hard corns are usually found on the tops of the toes and the sole of the foot. Soft corns are small, white patches of rubbery skin found only between the toes where the skin tends to be moist. They are caused by a combination of pressure and perspiration. Seed corns are tiny white dots that are usually painless. They tend to be associated with dry skin and are found on non-weight bearing areas of the foot, such as the arch. Corns can be prevented by good foot hygiene and wearing well-fitting shoes that do not cause friction. If corns are not painful, leave them alone. Otherwise, seek the advice of your doctor or a state registered chiropodist, or podiatrist.

Cramp

Cramp is a sudden intense pain due to a muscular spasm caused by prolonged contraction of the muscle tissue. It may be triggered by exercise, repetitive movements or holding an awkward position for a long time. Rubbing and stretching brings relief. Massage also helps to stimulate the circulation and removes waste products such as lactic acid that often lead to transient pain. Begin with a light pressure and gradually get firmer.

Diabetes

Diabetes can lead to various adverse side-effects including poor circulation and diminished sensation in the feet, and sometimes the hands. People with diabetes may have less awareness of temperature changes, rough surfaces and skin damage. As the sensation in the feet may be reduced, people with diabetes may not realize they have injured their feet, especially the soles. In a diabetic person, broken skin can take longer to heal and there is a poor response to infection, so a minor injury can quickly develop into a serious wound. If you have diabetes it is essential to maintain good foot hygiene, and have regular check-ups with your doctor and a state registered chiropodist, or podiatrist to prevent problems developing. Check your feet every day, using a mirror if necessary, and ensure you have no holes or rough areas in shoes, socks and tights.

Massage can help promote better circulation to the hands and feet, but it is important to seek professional advice first. When giving a massage, be aware of the temperature of the room and your depth of touch as your massage partner may not be able to give you feedback on feelings of cold or discomfort. Hand and foot mobility exercises will help – and follow the advice for boosting circulation on page 114.

Flat feet

Flat feet are sometimes referred to as dropped or fallen arches, which describes the condition well. Flat feet can affect posture and lead to knee and back problems. There is conflicting advice on whether or not to treat flat feet but there is a growing consensus that specialist adjustments to foot wear can reduce the risk of knee injuries and chronic lower back pain. Seek the advice of a doctor or a state registered chiropodist, or podiatrist.

Ganglions

These are small, painless lumps, usually pea-size but can be larger, caused by a build-up of fluid in the sheath surrounding a tendon. Ganglions are commonly found around the wrist and ankle joints. They are harmless and, if left alone, may disappear without treatment. If necessary, they can be surgically removed. Seek the advice of a doctor. Massage is not ruled out but work around the ganglion.

Hangnails

Hangnail are hard tags of skin that develops in the nail groove separate from the main nail plate. They usually occur when the cuticles becoming dry and stretched, or through injury to the nail root. Hangnails are also associated with nail biting or poor manicuring. The spike of nail looks unattractive, it can be painful and catch on clothes – especially tights. It is tempting to bite or pull on it, but this can lead to sore, broken skin or bleeding around the nail. To avoid hangnails, massage moisturizing cream into the cuticles and nails daily. Set time aside for a weekly manicure to care for your nails.

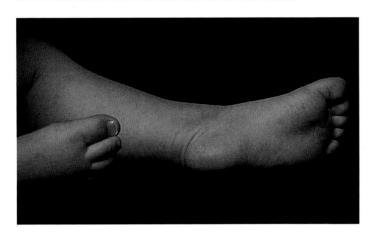

Ingrowing toenails

If a toenail grows into the surrounding skin and becomes embedded it is called an ingrowing toenail. The big toe is most commonly affected. If it has a sharp edge it can dig into the flesh and cause irritation, pain and even infection. An ingrowing toenail is tender to any pressure. It often occurs when the nails are cut too short, especially at the sides. However, it may be due to injury, pressure from tight shoes or excessive perspiration. Adolescent boys are particularly prone to ingrowing toenails. Prevent the condition by maintaining good foot hygiene, clipping toenails straight across and wearing shoes that do not squash the toes. If you have an ingrowing toenail, do not try to solve the problem yourself, go to your doctor or a state

registered chiropodist, or podiatrist. Do not massage if the area is painful and/or infected.

Nail biting

Nail biting, or onychophagy, to use the medical name, is a fairly common habit, especially among children. In severe cases the nails can bleed and look unsightly. It is a hard habit to break but worth the effort. Once you stop biting your nails they grow back normally. A good way of helping to break the habit is by caring for your hands and nails.

Have regular hand massages and manicures to improve hand and nail condition. When you see how much better they look, you'll be encouraged to stop biting your nails. Keep an emery board with you so you can file down any ragged edges that you might be tempted to chew.

Nail infections

These are most often caused by the fungus that causes athlete's foot, although can occur in the absence of athlete's foot. In some cases, however, the problem is due to a bacterial infection. The nail changes colour, often turning creamy white or yellow, and the underside becomes powdery and crumbles. Good hygiene is essential as the infection can be passed to finger nails. Nail infection can be a persistent condition. If it is caused by a fungus it usually responds to the same treatment as athlete's foot. But a bacterial nail infection requires specialist treatment. If the problem persists or becomes painful or irritating, see a doctor or a state registered chiropodist, or podiatrist. Do not massage until the condition has cleared up.

Osteoarthritis

Osteoarthritis, which is often simply called "arthritis", is common in people over 60. It is also known as the "wear and tear" complaint because it tends to affect the joints

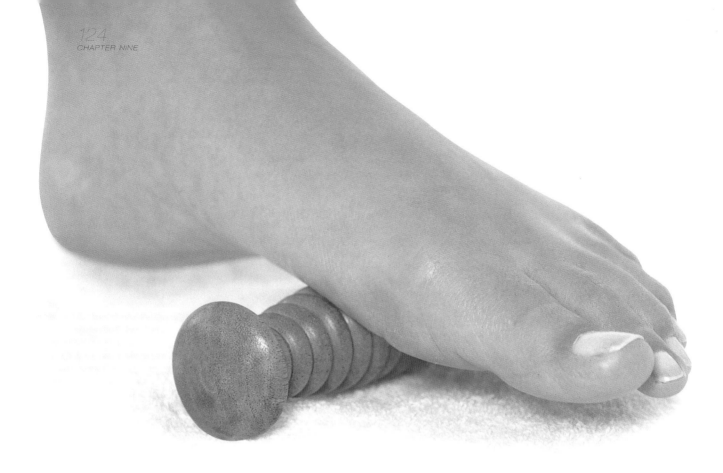

that have had most use over the years. The cartilage that lines the joints erodes and breaks up and the bone ends may begin to fuse, resulting in stiffness, inflammation and aching in the joints. The joints affected by osteoarthritis tend to take on a swollen and gnarled appearance. The big toe is often affected as so much pressure is placed on this joint every day, so well-fitting shoes are important. Your doctor or a state registered chiropodist, or podiatrist, will offer advice on coping with osteoarthritis and preventing further deterioration. Hand and foot mobility exercises are beneficial in helping to maintain movement in the joint – but never force it. Massage can help ease aches and pains and may give some temporary increase in mobility; but do not massage directly over a hot, swollen or inflamed joint as it creates heat that can aggravate the condition.

Rashes

Rashes are areas of skin that have become dry, inflamed or covered in spots. Eczema, psoriasis and dermatitis are common skin conditions that lead to itchy, red patches on the skin. The skin may become chapped in dry, cold wintry conditions. Non-contagious skin conditions usually benefit from massage – but check that your massage partner has consulted a doctor or skin specialist. Avoid if the disease is undiagnosed or you have any doubts. Massage with a suitable emollient will help moisturize skin, and boost the flow of blood and lymph to remove waste products and fight infection. Rashes should not be scratched as this may lead to broken skin which is open to infection.

Raynaud's disease

This is a condition in which the blood supply to the extremities, usually the fingers and toes, is interrupted because of constrictions in small blood vessels. It most often occurs as a result of extreme changes in temperature – too hot or too cold – or stress. It causes the fingers and toes to turn white and numb. As they get warmer and the blood starts flowing again, they go blue and then bright red. After an attack, they feel tingling and painful and it may take up to an hour before the feeling returns. Women are nine times more likely to suffer than men. Regular hand and foot massage and mobility exercises (see pages 116–9) help boost the circulation to the extremities and reduce the number of attacks. Take sensible precautions in winter, give up smoking and follow the tips for improving blood circulation on page 114. Wear well-fitting shoes and avoid holes in socks and tights. A pair of cotton gloves worn under woollen gloves help keep fingers warm.

Rheumatoid arthritis

Rheumatoid arthritis affects all the joints and muscles in the hands and feet, rather than a specific joint. It is a progressive disease that occurs when the immune system begins to attack the body's own tissues. Rheumatoid arthritis involves chronic inflammation of the connective tissue around a joint – and often affects the fingers and toes. The joints become inflamed, swollen and stiff, especially in the morning. Gentle hand and foot massage in the direction of the heart improve blood circulation and stimulate the flow of lymph to remove excess waste products and fluid from the area. Never massage directly over a hot, swollen or inflamed joint – keep your strokes above and below the joint. Hand and foot mobility exercises help to mobilize joints. Wear well-fitting shoes to accommodate any swelling and make regular visits to a state registered chiropodist, or podiatrist.

Sweatiness

Sweaty, smelly feet can be caused by a number of factors, including stress. The condition does not necessarily indicate any disease but, if allowed to continue, offers the ideal environment for fungal infection to take hold. Pay special attention to foot hygiene and go barefoot whenever safe and practical. Wear open-toed sandals in the summer. Wash your feet daily in warm water to which you have added two drops of geranium oil, a natural deodorant. Dry thoroughly and dust with an antifungal powder to keep the feet dry and absorb sweat. Massage helps calm nerves – but avoid if there are any signs of fungal infection. Do not wear the same pair of shoes every day and keep shoes in an area where they are exposed to fresh air.

Verrucae

Verrucae are caused by a virus that enters the body via broken skin. They are sometimes called "plantar warts" as they develop on the sole (plantar surface) of the foot. Verrucae vary in size and may be just 12 mm (about 1/2 in) across. They can be confused with corns but are usually more painful when pinched. The affected skin surface becomes rough and irregularly shaped with visible tiny black specks. They are highly contagious and thrive in moist, damp conditions. To avoid catching a verruca wear flip-flops in communal changing areas and have separate towels for each member of the family. Keep them covered to stop the spread of infection – and do not massage or pick at them. Most verrucae clear up within one to two years without treatment, but seek advice from your doctor or a state registered chiropodist, or podiatrist, if they cause discomfort or pain.

Warts

Warts are caused by the same viral infection as verrucae. They usually have a rough surface and grow in multiples – often around cuticles. Warts are harmless, but they are also contagious so keep them covered if you are in close contact with others – and do not massage or pick at them. Warts may go within a year or so without treatment, but if you have any concerns talk to your doctor.

Check your diet

A well-balanced diet, full of essential nutrients, is vital for maintaining the health of skin and nails. And it is never too late to start change eating habits because cells are constantly renewing themselves.

Top up fluid levels

Water is essential to good health – begin by drinking more fluid. Even mild dehydration will lead to dry skin, spots and brittle nails. We lose about 3 litres (over 5 pints) of water a day through perspiration, respiration and urination. Some of this is replaced by fluid in the food we eat, but not all. The recommended daily intake of water is around eight glasses, but you may need to drink a little

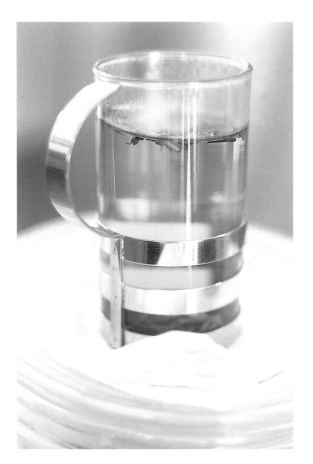

more in hot weather, after exercise and at times of stress or anxiety when there are higher demands on your body. Keep a bottle of water handy so that you can take sips throughout the day. Try drinking herbal teas, too. Camomile is very relaxing, nettle and dandelion are said to be good for nail growth, while ginger tea is reputed to stimulate blood circulation. Avoid excess alcohol which can dehydrate nails and skin. Alcohol also acts as a diuretic so you lose more fluid than you take in. A simple way of checking your hydration levels is to check the colour of your urine. It should be clear and pale. Dark yellow urine is a sign that you need to drink more water.

Essential nutrients

You should aim to eat at least five portions of fruit and vegetables every day, preferably organic, to boost fluid intake and ensure your body is getting sufficient vitamins and minerals. Vitamin C is vital for skin health, renewal and repair, keeping it firm and strong, and helps fight infection. Vitamin C is found in melon, pineapple, kiwi fruits, apples, fresh or dried apricots, green leafy vegetables and carrots. Vitamin A is also important for healthy skin and nails. Lack of Vitamin A causes a build up of dead skin leading to rough, dry, flaky skin. Good sources are carrots, watercress, cabbage and mangoes.

Zinc is essential for the growth, repair and renewal of cells. This mineral is needed for the formation of new, healthy skin and nail cells. Lack of zinc leads to flaky, dull skin and brittle nails and is associated with many skin problems. Zinc-rich foods include whole grains, nuts, seeds, lean meat and seafood. Another important mineral is iron, which is found in lean red meat, dark green vegetables, dried fruit and nuts. Lack of iron leads to pale skin, weak nails and sensitivity to cold.

Cell membranes are made from essential fats. Lack of essential fats causes rapid dehydration. If your skin and

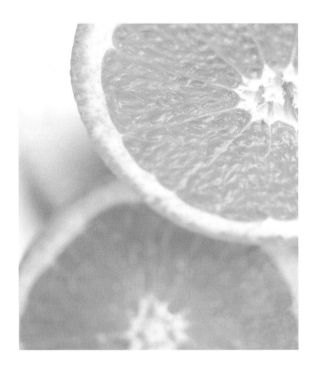

When breathing effectively, the movement comes from the diaphragm, not the chest. The diaphragm, a dome-like sheet of muscle that separates the chest from the abdomen, pushes downward to allow more air to flow deep down into the lungs. If you are aware that you tend to breathe too quickly or too shallowly, it is a good idea to practise controlling your breath. This is a good exercise to practise, especially during a stressful time. Notice how much more relaxed you feel afterward.

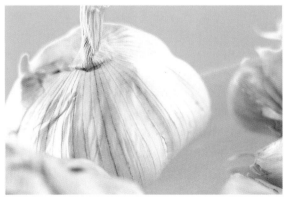

Breathing exercise

Set aside a few minutes. Lie comfortably on the floor. Breathe in deeply through your nose, drawing the breath right down to your abdomen. Hold this breath for a few moments, then allow it to flow out, slowly and gently. Imagine you are releasing your tension as your breath leaves your body. Repeat several times. To check you are doing this correctly, place one hand on your chest and the other on your abdomen. The hand on your chest should remain almost still while the hand on your abdomen rises and falls as you breathe in and out.

nails are very dry and flaky then increase your intake of essential fats. Good sources are oily fish, especially salmon, mackerel and sardines, and nuts and seeds. Essential fats are also found in unrefined cold-pressed oils such as sunflower, olive, sesame, walnut and corn – so use these to dress salads. Add garlic when cooking too – as this is useful for boosting the immune system to fight infection.

Breath of life

Your body relies on oxygen for good health. Fresh oxygen provides the energy you need for the proper functioning of every cell in the body – from the tips of your fingers to the ends of your toes. However, many people breathe poorly. The most common fault is fast, shallow breathing which means that the lungs are not being used to their full capacity. If breathing is not deep enough, inhaled air is not drawn down to the lower lungs where most of the blood circulates. Not only do you miss out on your full quota of oxygen, but the waste gas carbon dioxide is not being removed so efficiently.

fact

A good breathing technique can also help make your massage more effective – as it ensures that you have a full quota of oxygen to boost energy and concentration levels.

Index